I0420913

My Health and Fitness

Volume 1

39 Articles

By: Wade Yoder

Master Trainer - Fitness Nutrition Specialist

- Health & Fitness Columnist

Notes and Comments from News Publishers

"Wade Yoder has been offering expert health advice by way of weekly columns to readers of The Leader-Tribune, Citizen-Georgian and News Observer since 2012. Every week, Wade covers some aspect of health, diet, nutrition, exercise and lifestyle. His advice is always backed by science, often contrarian, sometimes controversial, but always informative, with an emphasis on giving readers tips they can put to immediate use and improve their health and fitness. The columns are filled with a passion for the health for our readers. We hear allot of good positive feed back from our readers that read and enjoy Wade's columns."
Judy Robinson/ Publisher
Victor Kulkosky/ Editor
The Leader Tribune
The Citizen Georgian
The News Observer

"Wade Yoder's articles are invaluable to the readers of The Taylor County News. They are extremely informative, providing very interesting and practical analogies to everyday life. Wade's quick wit draws the reader into the topic and his knowledge of health, fitness, and nutrition keeps them engaged until the end. I feel very blessed to provide Wade's valuable information to the readers."
Valori Moore ~ Publisher
Taylor County News

"Wade's column is one of the most read in The Georgia Post and people are always commenting on it as being informative."
Victoria Simmons/ Publisher
The Georgia Post and Byron Buzz

"I always enjoy your column in our local newspaper, The Citizen Georgian. You have a gift for physical fitness and holistic health in its entirety. I identify with a lot of the things you write about in your columns. Your articles help us realize that our choice eating habits, as well as healthy lifestyle changes, can be achieved through making small steps towards becoming a healthier and happier person from the inside out. I enjoy the wealth of knowledge you provide us with from week to week. Your readers feel and understand through your writing that goals can be attained in constructive ways by simply changing a habit, adopting a new mindset, and responding to life's challenges with greater wisdom and knowledge. Thank you for all that you do and keep the columns coming because I am a fan! And I think you are a very excellent and informative writer!"
Sharonda West~ Publisher
The Citizen and Georgian

Note from the author: I value the opinions from ones in the medical field as well and have benefitted from my uncle Richard and aunt Martha's views on things from a medical perspective. The following two notes are from them in regard to my published articles, and newsletters.

Martha Kauffman, RN, BSN

Augusta, GA

 I am always impressed with Wade's newsletters and his knowledge of how the body works; his helpful suggestions of how to properly exercise, and also how proper nutrition is so important to maintain and support the immune system.

Richard Kauffman, M.D.

Atlanta, GA

 Have you ever wondered, "why is there so much cancer in our country as compared to some other countries in the world?" For instance, here in the United States the rate of cancer is approximately 450 per 100,000 persons that have some kind of cancer at any given moment in time. Compare that to Niger where the rate is only 63.4 per 100,000 persons. Why is there such a huge difference? Diet and lifestyle!

Wade is right on when it comes to expressing his ideas on how to attain and maintain a healthy mind and body. He will give you pertinent facts from his research to back up what he states in his opinions. You will find his readings to be insightful and full of great suggestions for living life to its fullest potential.

I have known Wade for many years since I am his uncle. I have watched him grow from an inquisitive child into an astonishing inquisitive and capable adult who has a deep passion for living life to its fullest potential. You will enjoy reading his perspectives on how life can be healthy, vigorous and enjoyable.

Kauffman, et al, The Frequency of Protease and Reverse Transcriptase Gene Mutations and
    Corresponding Drug Resistance Profile in Primary Care Settings in Atlanta, GA.

Presented at the 36th Annual Meeting of Infectious Diseases Society of America – November 12 – 15, 1998 – Denver, CO (Abstract # 469-Sa)

Kauffman, et al, Viral Load Response Following Genotypic Antiretroviral Resistance Testing (GART) In Primary Care Settings in Atlanta, GA.

Presented at the 14th International Congress on Drug Therapy in HIV Infection, November 8 – 12, 1998 – Glasgow, Scotland (Abstract # 64)

Introduction

Have you ever wondered why health, fitness, prevention of chronic disease and premature aging has become so complicated? It's largely due to the industrialization of things that detract us from the basic fundamentals of health and fitness.

Example: losing weight shouldn't cost you money it should save you money! We store a lot of calories in our body fat and our body knows very well how to extract them during a calorie deficit, especially if we get our blood sugar level low enough.

My Health and Fitness Volume 1 is a mix of 39 articles on burning body fat naturally, building muscle without supplements, increasing mobility and capability, prevention of chronic disease and premature aging. These fundamentals have not changed and the confusion and hype surrounding them is used is not for your benefit. I have been in the health club business since 1991 and have seen a lot of fads and hype come and go, but not without taking a lot of consumer monies with them.

Dedicated to: the discouraged, the scared, the financially strapped, the hurting, the confused, the frustrated and last but not least, the ones who feel that spending a major amount of their life in doctor's office waiting rooms and endless diagnosis's is the new norm...

This book and series is dedicated to helping everyone I can to realize the power of the body's own resources when given the simple basics that it craves, such as the body's capability to fight premature aging and chronic disease, by formulating its own drugs through the power of the immune system.

Health, fitness, muscle building and weight loss should not be looked at as something that costs a lot of money. Our health and fitness is adaptive to the habits we adopt.

If this book helps make your path to health and fitness an easier less complicated one, then my mission is accomplished~ Wade Yoder

"Ask why, and ask it again five more times, until all the artifice is stripped away, and you need up with the intellectually honest answer." ~Andy Grove

For Thou didst form my inward parts: Thou didst cover me in my mother's womb. I will give thanks unto thee, for I am fearfully and wonderfully made ~ Psalm 139, 13-14

Table of Contents

6 THINGS TO ASK YOURSELF IF YOU'RE NOT FEELING WELL

There are some very important questions we should ask ourselves when we're not feeling well.

These are the basics we need to physiologically keep our bodies functioning properly. The next in importance is consistency and quality of each of these habits. Most chronic diseases and issues will either gradually or in some cases rapidly straighten themselves out (without medical diagnostics, medicine or continued medical therapy) when we give our body the healthy things it craves.

Questions I need to ask myself if I'm not feeling well

1. Am I getting plenty of clean air?

2. Am I getting plenty of clean water?

3. Am I getting a balanced diet?

4. Am I getting out into the open air and sunshine?

5. Am I getting enough activity/exercise?

6. Am I getting deep rest?

 If I do not feel good about the amount, consistency or the quality that I'm getting of any of the above, I may have the diagnosis of why I'm not feeling well.

AGING = OXIDATION AND OXIDATION = AGING

If you can figure out how to slow down the oxidation process in your body, you can slow down the aging process as well as decreasing chronic disease formation.

We need food to sustain life, but metabolism of these calories into energy, and the extraction of nutrients, (as well as our exposure to other things in life such as food and environmental toxins), creates oxidation. This is a byproduct of all the processes that are happening in our body and its systems. Our body works like a factory and if we don't help it to release the toxic byproducts, these toxins will build up and cause us problems, (imagine closing the smokestack on a factory).

Water, sweat, antioxidants, muscular movement and our waste elimination system are like a drainage system that helps us cleanse out and get rid of these toxins that cause aging and disease. If we don't get these toxins out of us, an oxidative process will begin causing constant inflammatory conditions that can lead to premature aging and disease!

Example: if our car gets a deep scratch, it will eventually begin to oxidize (if not taken care of), and will manifest itself as rust. In our body however this rusting can be translated to chronic inflammation, which is the source that almost all chronic diseases get their energy from. This inflammation is sort of like a clump of rust that continues to draw energy to itself and if the root cause of the rust is not stopped, the effected area will continue to deteriorate until it is ruined. In much the same way, if whatever is causing inflammation is not stopped and this oxidation continues, a medical specialist will eventually be able to diagnose and give a name for whatever it has prevailed itself to be, whether it's a diseased body part, or a systemic disease affecting other parts of the body.

Free radicals: when we allow toxins to build up or continue to enter our body, free radicals are formed that cause oxidative damage to our eyes, skin, muscle, fat, vital organs, bones, ligaments, tendons etc. And though these body parts may still work, they hurt more and operate in a less efficient and aged manner.

 Free radicals need electrons, so they steal electrons away from healthy surrounding cells, turning them into free radicals as well. This is how oxidation and disease grows in the body and whether systemic or in clusters, this can be the beginning of a chronic condition and if not neutralized can eventually turn into a chronic disease.

 Immune system, free radicals, and oxidation: our immune system sometimes uses the oxidative process to kill viruses and bad bacteria, (this is actually a good thing), but if we continue to be exposed to the things that are triggering this reaction, we get what we know as chronic inflammation. This oxidative and inflammatory process leads to disease and premature aging in the areas it is happening at!

Example: we oft times worry about our skin aging as well as the smoothness and firmness of our fatty areas. The aging process of either is quite simple, oxidative stress causes the collagen in our skin to lose its elasticity, which in turn creates wrinkles. Oxidation also creates aged pitted looking fat we call cellulite and cellulite is to fat like a wrinkle is to the skin.

What we can do: since oxidation is a byproduct of free radicals, and antioxidants neutralize them, doesn't it make sense to increase (antioxidant rich) fruits and vegetables in our diet? If you raise your own fruits and vegetables, (even though it may not have an attractive nutritional label or come in a pretty container) you have the best source at your fingertips for increasing your antioxidant levels!

If your only access is fruits and vegetables passed through modern logistic systems, I highly recommend fruit and vegetable extract powders to supplement your diet. However, research the company, and the science behind the product.

In a nutshell: drinking adequate water every day along with a good diet that includes a variety of fruits and vegetables (they are the best source for anti-oxidants), along with sweat and proper waste elimination, will help you fight the oxidation process in the body.

Try this natural cleanse: Eat only fruits, vegetables, nuts, and beans for 5-7 days along with 1/2 your bodyweight in oz. of water. Fruits need to be eaten the early part of the day to assist with the body's natural detox time period, which is for about 6 hours after waking. I highly recommend drinking unsweetened lemon water from fresh squeezed lemons during this time period as well.

Also use healthy oils, (like olive oil on salads, or supplement with fish oil caps), this will assist in waste removal and will help keep energy levels steady as well.

Premature aging and disease is an accumulation of oxidation that simply builds up enough to become a diagnosable problem. Lets live an Anti-Oxidation lifestyle!

SARCOPENIA = AGE RELATED MUSCLE LOSS

Sarcopenia from the Greek meaning **poverty of flesh** is the degenerative loss of skeletal muscle mass and strength associated with aging.

 The study of sarcopenia really intrigued me when I read the book Bio Markers, on how "You can control the aging process." A lot of the normal signs that we have accepted as being a part of the aging process, (such as slowing metabolism, muscle loss, skeletal and cardiovascular weaknesses), often have more to do with inactivity and diet causing muscle loss, then it does with aging. Research shows that one of the first signs of the aging process is a loss of protein (muscle) in the body. The two main contributing factors to this loss of muscle (sarcopenia) are simply, inactivity and diet. So it's quite simple to slow down and even reverse the symptoms of aging, through our diet and lifting weights. The body builds itself up to counter increased demands!

Over the past 20 plus years in the fitness business, I have seen a lot of difference (in how the aging process is offset) when individuals adapt a consistent, active lifestyle that keeps both mind and body challenged. Challenging our body and mind to new things can really go a long way in helping us to sidestep mental and physical deterioration in our latter years!

This is a quote from Miriam Nelson, a professor of nutrition at Tufts University; "A 70-year-old active individual is probably younger from a biomarker standpoint - muscle strength, balance, body composition, blood pressure, cholesterol levels - than a 40-year-old inactive person." This means we can literally turn back the clock on things that have aged our body, through simple rejuvenating changes to our lifestyle!

Preventing sarcopenia: we can counter the shrinking muscle mass, decreased bone density, and weakening of our cardiovascular system, using two primary tools, (exercise and our diet) and in many cases can make things much better. When you feel and look better then you did in 5-10-15-

and even 20 years, it can really make you feel like you're winding back the clock! There are some simple guides below to protect you against sarcopenia and shrinkage of life...

How muscle grows: the muscle building process is simply a response to muscle straining against a heavier load then it is used to. This causes small microscopic tears in the muscle fibers, which in turn places an order to the rebuilding system of our body, to patch up these little micro tears with amino acids (from the protein in our diet), thus building a new and stronger muscle!

Our body breaks down protein into amino acids to rebuild and patch up our broken down muscle, and this is the reason we need to increase the protein in our diet, especially when we exercise or do things that cause physical strain to our bodies.

Bone density: though bone density is not a part of the meaning of sarcopenia, our reversal of sarcopenia (muscle building or rebuilding) can have a direct impact on new gains in bone density as well. Just like skeletal muscle, when greater workloads are applied to bones, joints, and tendons, our body recognizes the need for stronger bones and connective tissue.

Cardiopulmonary strength: when we increase our muscle strength, it should also have a direct impact on creating better blood flow as well as strengthening our vital organs and the overall physiological functions of our body. When we have better flow of nutrients to the various parts of our body, things will start waking up like the plants in a garden do after a nice spring rain!

Our body builds what we tell it to, but also shrinks what we tell it to, and we speak these instructions to our body through activity or inactivity as well as what we choose for food and drink. We not only are what we eat, we also become what we do with what we eat!

We oft times complain about health, physical appearance and physical capabilities, when we're actually the one telling our body how to behave through our lifestyle habits.

When we place a consistent demand (with slow increases over time), on our skeletal muscle as well as our cardiovascular system we can prevent a lot of this lifestyle related shrinkage of muscle size, strength and endurance. The cardiovascular (endurance) part seems to gradually improve, as we're able to do these exercises more vigorously.

Resistance training with free weights: this helps increase strength and balance. Do exercises that involve several muscle groups (compound movements). Compound movements get your muscles trained to work together as they become stronger. Start off with gradual increases and chart your progress. This really adds up when multiplied by the month and then by the year(s)!

Nutrition: Increase protein and fat intake, (this increases our capability to build muscle and hormones), eat more dark colored vegetables, and eat your fruits in the early part of the day. Avoid starches and sugars, especially with high fat meals. Include plenty of nuts and beans in your diet.

 When demand is placed against it, our body is designed to become stronger to accommodate these new stressors, whether in muscular, skeletal or in cardiovascular fitness!

Staying strong helps match your health span to your lifespan.

INTERMITTENT FASTING (IF)

For those that are not familiar with the term, intermittent fasting is just going for **intermittent periods of fasting** with no food, and working them into your lifestyle.

This can be either once a week or several times a week and usually lasts anywhere from 12-24 hours. This is an inexpensive way to drop weight (burn fat) over time without worrying about losing muscle tissue, or worrying about which fat burner or diet will work the best. Stored fat is like our survival pantry with cans of stored food, (they both supply us with calories when we are in need). So next time someone tries to convince you to spend money to lose weight, remember that it's a little like paying someone to burn up the supply of food that you spent both time and money storing up in your pantry.

The way I do the intermittent fast (IF): after my last meal of the day, I simply go into the following day, extending the time of the first meal or snack. I do not break-the-fast (this is the meaning of breakfast) until either afternoon or early evening. This lowers the level of insulin produced which in turn will signal release of calories from stored fat, to take the place of the ones we're not getting through our stomach.

A calorie deficit in our stomach will signal for the release of stored calories (fat). And since there are around 3500 calories in a pound of fat, by dropping about 18-24 hours of normal food intake, your deficit can really cut into a pound of fat! I like to do this once a week, but depending on the amount of fat you're wanting to lose, you could do it up to 3 separate times a week without worrying about muscle loss.

How much can you burn in a day: on average, a person needs to add an extra zero to their bodyweight to get a minimum number of calories burned in a days time, at rest.

Example: a 160 lb. person would need 1600 calories base line, without figuring daily physical activity. So if a 160 lb. person skipped eating for 24 hours, they should burn at least a half-pound of stored energy (fat).

The idea behind intermittent fasting: getting insulin levels low, (triggers the release of body fat as an energy source). When we take in sugary and starch filled foods and snacks foods, our body recognizes a fuel entering the system that can be dangerous if left in the blood, so it releases insulin to not only help the body safely remove it from the blood and into our cells, but to also turn off the fat burning process until its job is done. The presence of insulin in the blood simply shuts down the fat burning process.

Stretching out the fat burning effect: an intake of proteins and fats (from meats, eggs, nuts, beans) along with dark colored vegetables work really well if you want to extend the fat burning effect but avoid going into starvation mode.

Warning: if you go low calorie or complete calorie restriction for too long, your body will think it is starving and will accommodate the lower food intake by lowering your metabolism, (it does this by breaking down muscle for energy). Oft times when someone gets on appetite suppressants, they will stay low calorie for too long, causing the body to go into a catabolic state, (it does this to protect us during times of starvation). However, you can trick your body into continuing to burn fat, by having an in-between cheat meal and refueling the hungry muscle cells before once again diving back into a fat burning calorie deficit!

Always remember, whether intermittent fasting or low calorie, simply cycling your calorie intake up and down with high and low energy output days is a good way to control our weight. In other words, don't put racing fuel in a slow moving vehicle!

Drink plenty of water, as this is your only source of hydration during periods of fasting.

ME VS. HEALTHCARE

Early detection by the medical field, should have never attempted to step into the shoes of prevention, it is incapable of yielding the same benefits.

Navigating healthcare and healthcare options is something we have been hearing a lot about and it can be unnerving to say the least! We have a huge aging population which will be stretching our healthcare system and capabilities to the max and it's enough to give all of us concern as to what kind of care we can expect if we ourselves or family need healthcare services.

It really impacted me when I read a September 2012 article in the Wall Street Journal- where it said that there are enough people that die each week from medical mistakes to fill 4 jumbo jets. This does not include the ones with temporary or lifetime complications from medical mistakes. As the system gets loaded with more and more patients due to our aging population, we need to consider that quality of care may decline due to wait times, and less time for individual care by the healthcare professional.

We have overused and abused medical access for years and have grown a dependency that we need to assess and possibly back off from. We can decrease our dependency oft times by changing some lifestyle habits and we can track down some answers simply by asking ourselves a few simple questions,

1. What have I been doing wrong?

2. What have I not been doing right?

3. How long has 1 or 2 been going on?

4. What can I do to correct this?

Asking ourselves these questions and answering them honestly can put us on track for decreasing our dependency on others for our health.

Self diagnostic questions we can ask ourselves: have I been getting adequate water - have I been getting plenty of activity and exercise -

have I been eating a balanced diet with plenty of fruits and vegetables every day, and have I been getting good deep sleep?

We have an internal doctor (our immune system) that works 24x7x365 and it isn't practicing medicine- it knows exactly what's wrong and what it needs to repair and rejuvenate us with. Most of the time all this internal system is asking from us is a better diet, more water, more activity and better rest.

1. When you feel fine and your doctor is constantly trying to get you to come back for checkups (remember this is a business to them), but for you it's subjecting yourself to a gathering place of sick people many times unnecessarily.

2. When it comes to our medicine(s) we need to know the purpose of each and every one.

3. Learn all the side effects of each medicine, before using it.

4. If you're on medicine(s), question yourself and your doctor, to see if there is anything in your lifestyle that you can change or add to lessen the need for the medicine over time?

 If we can change our thought pattern from how we will be able to access healthcare, to a more defensive play of how can I keep myself from needing the healthcare system, (we can save ourselves a lot of down time as well as exposure to other pathogens etc. while we are in doctor' offices, hospitals and waiting rooms). This helps create healthcare independence and that is much better then healthcare dependence!

CUTTING THROUGH THE CLUTTER

 The basic principles of health, fitness and nutrition pretty much stay the same. Much of the confusion from health, fitness and medical marketing, has more to do with selling more medicine, supplements, gym memberships, fitness equipment and programs then it does your actual health and fitness!

 There is lots of health, fitness and medical information available and it can be very easy to let these additions take away from the basics. And just like our vehicle, if we spend too much time adding accessories, it can take our attention off of basic upkeep. And we know quite well, if we don't do basic upkeep and maintenance on our vehicles we most likely will have to repair things that could've been avoided.

1. Eating a variety of healthy foods, stay away from man made, processed foods as much as possible. Eating a variety of colors etc. helps keep our blood built up with a variety of nutrients and (these are the tools your inner mechanic uses to fix things and keep your system strong).

2. Stay active, every day and (make sure the muscles you use for pulling and pushing in your upper body get used as well).

3. Stay hydrated- Drink 1/2 your body weight in ounces of water.

4. Get deep rest, (don't eat or drink things that will stimulate energy or will drive your heart rate up because of heavy digestion).

5. When on any medicine, the number one priority should be to lessen the usage over time, unless the condition cannot be remedied with good diet, exercise, plenty of water and rest.

  Hippocrates said "Let food be thy medicine and medicine be thy food." He said this around 450-350 BC and he's still right, over 2000 years later. What is the value of paying a mechanic for a diagnostic test to see what is wrong with our car if we already knew that we were putting junk fuel in the tank? Lots of money is made in the field of medicine and nutrition from confusion.

Don't let anything distract you from the basics coming first; everything else is additions and trimmings!

WHY IS FOOD THAT WAS GOOD BEFORE, BAD NOW AND VICE VERSA?

Have you ever wondered why after 50+ years a food that was once thought as good for you suddenly becomes bad, or a food that was once thought of as not so good comes back into favor?

What they often fail to talk about is the supporting dietary factors that may cause these same foods to have a negative health effect now when they didn't before.

Example: studies have shown the consumption of red meats lead to an increase in heart disease, cancer and death. They failed to note what we tend to eat with red meat now vs. before when we had fresh plenty of fresh fruits and vegetables in our diets, instead of consuming loads of sugars and starches with the red meats. They also failed to note the potential toxic effects of large insulin spikes when consuming meats or other high fat foods with sugars and starches!

 A diet with lots of antioxidant rich fruits, vegetables, not only assists us in detoxifying our body from the digestion of fats and proteins, the fiber helps move the meat along in our digestive tract. There's a big difference when we eat white bread, fries, sodas, sweet tea, or sugar loaded deserts with meat or other high fat foods.

 It would probably help if we form a mental picture, of the big sticky glob that we put into our stomach when we eat the above listed food combinations and subsequently what our digestive tract has to go through to process what it needs and then to eliminate the waste.

  If we eat a good blend of proteins, healthy fats, and complex carbohydrates from lean meats, eggs, nuts, beans, fruits, vegetables, grains, berries along with plenty of water, it will go a long way toward balancing out our needs, and in keeping us feeling good inside and out. **Remember-** our bodies really don't like certain components of processed foods (or when we blend a bunch of other stuff into and onto the things it recognizes as food). These things can irritate the lining of our digestive system causing a puffy immune reaction to happen. When our digestive tract is inflamed, it can make it more permeable (leaky gut) and when this happens, it can cause all kinds of autoimmune disorders.

Processed foods not only take a food away from its original form, it oft times involves adding in things that decrease the quality of the original food.

Example: when the squash becomes squash casserole, tomatoes become ketchup, peaches become cobblers and apples become apple pie. I'm not saying these are all bad foods it's the continuous or over usage of these processed foods and condiments will yield cumulative results that we don't like, in our health and our physical condition, if they're a large part of our diet.

The more we can stick with single item foods such as eggs, oatmeal and other whole grains, nuts, beans, raw milk, healthy oils, fruits, vegetables, non processed meats etc. the better off we are. And lets not forget drinking water, (without the additives that produce a cheapened end product)!

You don't even have to get super strict, you can simply keep plenty of the good foods around to add into your daily diet, and it will go a long way toward balancing out and trimming out the bad in our diet.

We are and will become a product of, what we eat and drink.

LOCALLY GROWN

There's a lot of value in eating locally grown fruits and vegetables whenever you can. Growing some of your own food or having a small garden is really good and besides the healthy fruits and vegetables, knowing how to grow at least some of your own food is a great thing!

When fruits and vegetables are picked and sold locally, they can be picked at the ripened stage. I like to think of the fruit or vegetable at the ripened stage as the point when the plant, tree or vine is finished with its project. Have you ever noticed how willing the plant, tree or vine is to turn it loose once it has finished its work vs. when the fruit or vegetable hasn't ripened? Once it's ripened, the plant is finished with its nutritious project.

We know that locally produced honey can help with allergy symptoms in your particular area, since the bees make it with pollen from this same area, and using this honey seems to help you become more resistant to the pollen. Have you ever noticed that certain fruits and vegetables grow really well in some regions and not in others? We are also exposed to these same conditions, so when we have the opportunity to eat the foods that nature packages for us from this area, it just may be exactly the designer foods we need, to help us do better as well.

 Fruits and vegetables are loaded with vitamins, minerals and phytonutrients.

Example: there are over 400 known and named nutrients in an apple, plus many more that are unnamed. I like to think of fruits and vegetables as nature's multi-vitamin package and when grown in the area you're in, it becomes a multi-vitamin perfectly designed and packaged by The Master Blender for the people in that area.

  I don't want to completely take away from the value of adding in vitamin and mineral supplementation, especially for a person that does not get 5-7 servings a day, but for the most part we can trust nature's multi-vitamin and mineral packages from fruits and vegetables any day over man made multi-vitamins and minerals! These are the foods that supply the 1000's of nutrients that help us fight disease!

YOU'RE NEVER TOO OLD FOR EXERCISE AND FITNESS!

This was a birthday article I wrote in honor of my oldest member. When someone is strong and fit going into their 80's and 90's, I like to learn everything I can about what makes them tick!

I would like to start out by wishing my oldest member Bell Vinson a Happy 92nd Birthday, May 30, 1920! His strong faith in God, physical strength, agility and mental keenness are a real inspiration to us at the gym.

Here are a few tidbits of wisdom from Mr. Vinson;

1. On Mental and Physical Health: "I think life - I do not think death, as a man thinketh so shall he be" (this also includes the ladies).

2. We control our thoughts on a conscious level, which affects our subconscious mind, and our subconscious controls our body on a cellular level.

3. I keep my mind wrapped around big things

4. Embrace changes, don't resist it, and be receptive to the new generation's way of doing things.

5. On Diet: When I asked him about diet, he simply said, "When I get hungry I eat."

I could get long winded on why I think the above basics have worked so well for Mr. Vinson, but for what I have seen and what I know of Mr. Vinson, the best way I know to sum it up is

1. His love and faith in God, which relieves a lot of stress in a person's life.

2. His interest in life and his love for the people in it.

3. Keeping his mind wrapped around big things showed me that (even though he is a retired pastor) he believes in remaining a student of life and trying to learn new things to keep the mind healthy and sharp.

4. I have to admit that when he said what he did about diet, it shocked me. I was hoping to learn about a special diet that he used, or at the least certain foods that he really liked, instead it was simply, that he eats when his body tells him it needs food.

Mr. Vinson is a true example of how well the body works when you have internal health first, (both spiritual and mental), continue challenging your mind to learn new things, adapt to changing times, stay active and listen to what your body needs.

Remember that healthy habits help turn back the clock on aging, no matter what the number is! Happy Birthday Mr. Bell Vinson!!!

YOU CANNOT OUT EXERCISE A BAD DIET!

About 70% of our physical shape depends on what we consume. Its easy to plan to hit the exercise routine a little harder the next day, and get back on a diet the following week, (when we're full of food), but unless we lower our caloric intake the next few meals or the next day, we simply burn the current day's calories that we consume. These excess calories we took in the day before will be turned into stored energy and this is what inflates our fat cells.

We can very easily create a calorie deficit for the current day, especially if we know we over did it the night before, by simply not eating for a while the next day, or by eating very little. I like to do an intermittent fast (IF) about once a week after having a good splurge meal the evening before. I do this by going for about 18-24 hours before I eat again, (sometimes I'll have a protein shake or something very light).

When eating less, you will usually feel tired and when your body is fixing to shift energy pathways, (you may feel a little weak). However once your insulin level is lowered in your blood from not having to be there for delivery of food nutrients (especially sugars), your body can then trigger the release of energy from your fat cells. Before this triggers the release of fat for energy, insulin in you blood, has to be low, (this means stay away from sugars and starches).

This is the way to lower the amount of energy substance inside our fat cells, and this is what we know as burning fat for energy! Burning the energy inside our fat cells is like letting the air out of a lot of balloons and being able to fit the shrunk up balloons back into a little box. What makes fat cells get big is the amount of energy we ourselves decide to keep stored in them.

Most of us don't want a lot of extra body fat, but the thing to keep in mind is its simply stored energy that we need to figure out how to release. Sugary foods, drinks, and foods that can convert to sugar rapidly are the BIG culprits in not only causing weight gain, but also in preventing the fat cells from releasing their energy!

 Eating the right foods and controlled portion sizes so as to stimulate your body's natural fat burn process between meals and toning your muscles, (all over your body), will turn your body into a natural fat and calorie burning machine!

Take away: Sugar (enough to cause a blood sugar spike) is not only bad for your health; it also turns off the fat burning process in your body!

YOUR KITCHEN CAN BE YOUR FAT BURNING TOOL CHEST

Dietary Thermogenesis and the Thermic Effect Of Food.

In reality, ALL foods are thermogenic because the body must use energy to digest them. This is known as the thermic effect of food (TEF) or the specific dynamic action of food. However, not all foods have the same thermic effect. Some are very mushy and easily absorbed.

Example: A grilled chicken breast, sweet potato and broccoli vs. a small Oreo Blizzard btw they are my weakness! The plate of food and the Oreo blizzard would probably be around the same amount of calories, but the calorie load from the blizzard would hit your bloodstream much faster then the big plate of food would. When you consume a sugar, whether in food, drinks, or starchy foods, the sugars will be ready to use as energy very rapidly and if you're not active, insulin (if working properly) will help remove the extra sugar from our blood and will store it in our fat cells as stored energy. This is what makes our fat cells expand.

Foods that are not processed from their original state (fruits, vegetables, nuts, lean meats etc.) usually take longer to breakdown and thus give you a longer sustained stream of energy. Our body will burn more calories if we choose foods that break down more slowly.

The most thermogenic food is lean protein from solid foods, especially the following:

- Chicken breast
- Turkey breast
- Game meats (venison, elk, etc.)
- Bison, buffalo
- Very lean red meat such as top round and lean sirloin (grass fed is especially nutritious)
- Most types of fish

- Shellfish and other seafood

Other foods to use in your kitchen arsenal

- Eggs
- Kale
- Mushrooms
- Walnuts
- Rolled oats
- Sweet potato
- Avocado
- Hemp seeds
- Black beans
- Wild salmon
- Pears
- Dark colored vegetables

3-Step Formula To Put Together A Fat-Burning Meal:

STEP 1: Select a green vegetable or fibrous vegetable such as asparagus, green beans, broccoli,

Brussels sprouts, cauliflower and salad vegetables.

STEP 2: Combine one or several of the above with a lean protein (previously mentioned above).

STEP 3: The lean protein and fibrous carbohydrates form the foundation of your fat burning meal. From there, add natural starchy carbohydrates or grains such as brown rice, oats, or sweet potatoes - use these in the amount of energy you're needing to replace or to supply you for the next few hours. Fruit is also okay, but focus even more on the green and fibrous vegetables and do NOT eat fruits and vegetables together, (this is bad for digestion).

Fat Fighter Foods add these to your kitchen arsenal: beans, brown rice, quinoa and whole-grain pasta. These are considered resistant-starch foods. Resistant starch is a type of carbohydrate that resists digestion in the small intestine, gives you a feeling of fullness, raises metabolism, and controls blood sugar and cravings.

Take Away: About 70% of our shape depends on what we eat and drink so if we can surround ourselves with a good variety of healthy foods, we can satisfy food cravings and stay on track with our health and fitness.

THE PURPOSE OF INDIVIDUAL FOOD NUTRIENTS

It is very important to have a balanced diet that gives us the macro and micronutrients we need. This is what helps us keep our motor running smoothly!

Protein: We need protein for strengthening and repairing our muscles and organs. When stressed out with a heavy workload, the stressed part(s) of our body goes through a temporary breakdown process. Our body takes protein and breaks it down into amino acids or as I like to call it "muscle patch paint" and when it goes through this repair process it has then strengthened, toned or reinforced that particular stressed area of the body. Whether for bodybuilding, power lifting, sports or simply activities of daily living (ADL), protein is very necessary to sustain life!

Fat: We need this for hormone production, and to lubricate our system. It is also a condensed energy that burns much steadier then sugar. Our brain is mostly made up of fat, and even though we tend to dislike it if we have too much of it on our body, it is a macronutrient that we very much need as a part of our diet and is very essential for life sustenance.

Carbohydrates and Sugars: These are good for quick energy. Complex carbohydrates are better in that they breakdown slower into glucose, but if you need a faster source of energy, a more simple carbohydrates or something that has some sugar in it (usually most foods/drinks that taste sweet) can be okay for the times that you're running on empty and need something fast. You see it's when we don't burn these sugars as they enter our blood and become available as energy, that blood sugar and obesity problems start. Our insulin has a duty to clear the blood of high glucose levels and will cart the unused sugars/glucose off to be store in our fat cells. And this is what makes our fat cells oft times have an appearance we don't like. Fat cells are simply reserve holding tanks for energy, and it's up to us how big we make them or how small we shrink them.

Anti-Oxidants (vitamins and minerals):
These are what help protect us from disease as well as keeping such things as fluids in balance. When we keep our blood rich in a variety of antioxidants it works like safety armor for our skin, eyes, muscle, vital organs etc. When we don't have an adequate daily supply of these in our diet, it leaves us exposed to oxidation (rusting of our body), which we know as disease and premature aging.

Our best source for these is not some exotic berry from down in the Amazon that some network marketing company is trying to say is the next best thing, but simply the fruits and vegetables you can find at your local farmers market, roadside stand or can grow in your own back yard. The arrays of colors are nutrients and there are thousands of phytonutrients in a good variety of fruits and vegetables. These are the multi-vitamin and mineral packages designed for the people in the areas they are grown.

Remember its not just about eating healthy foods, but also in eating a good variety of healthy foods from the above listed categories, so that our body can pick and pull the tools of nutrition that it needs and just like a good mechanic will do its best to keep your vehicle running smoothly.

DON'T WAIT ON THE DOCTOR

We oft times wait to go to a doctor to simply let him or her diagnose a summary of bad habits over the past several days, weeks, months or even years that has finally accumulated enough to where it is diagnosable.

Example: our body fights cancer everyday. It's through life's series of ups and downs with our immune system, exposures to environmental toxins, our diets, inabilities of our immune system to discover cancer (mostly diet related) and quite simply our body's inability to expel toxins faster then they accumulate that it gets to a point that it becomes a diagnosable disease.

These toxins are responsible for forming the free radicals in our body that cause oxidation. Simply put, free radicals and oxidation is a rusting of our body. This can cause anything from the collagen in our skin losing its elasticity and forming wrinkles to the more serious chronic diseases such as cancer, heart disease etc. These toxins affect the DNA of our cells and this is what gives instructions on how to build the new generation of cells that our body continues to build everyday. When the blueprint gets corrupted it builds the cells differently and causes our looks to change more rapidly as we get older. If someone has strong DNA they are much more apt to age gracefully.

Our body has ways of getting rid of the bad stuff if we assist it in simple things such as: getting plenty of fresh air, working up a sweat, drinking plenty of water, and a diet rich in fruits and vegetables.

Getting proactive now with prevention instead of reactive when we feel symptoms of disease will lessen our dependency and reliance on the healthcare system. Many symptoms have a lifestyle offset and if we can find the offset and correct what it is we are lacking in, most times we can increase our body's capacity for fighting the disease.

We have replaced death by infectious disease with death by chronic disease, which is mostly diet, and lifestyle related, which means we can do something about it! **We live too short and die too long**!

Take away: Help preserve or rebuild health by adapting simple healthy lifestyle habits by staying hydrated with water, staying active, getting good quality rest, clean air, sunshine and a balanced diet.

 These healthy habits done with consistency will help us lead a full healthy life until our Maker turns our cellular switches off, so lets go out with a BANG!!!

HEALTH AND INDEPENDENCE

We all know that the opposite of independence is dependence and we do not like the feeling it gives us when we lose our freedom or our self-reliance. When we lose our independence we become subjected to someone else's way of doing things, puts us on their timing and makes us subject to their choices and decisions.

Staying healthy and strong can help us in maintaining our independence in our Activities of Daily Living (ADL's), it also can decrease or possibly eliminate medicine, we can spend less time out of our lives in doctor's offices and the list goes on and on.

There are two things that we should ask ourselves:

1. What is inhibiting my health now?

2. What have I done, or what am I doing that may potentially put my health at risk in the future?

We start losing our independence when we start increasing our dependence on others, but we can oft times regain our independence if we continue to at least try to do the things today that we want to be able to do or continue to do tomorrow.

Take Away: When we know the issues that we face with our health and what we want to prevent, we can then ask ourselves, "what can we do now and in the future that will help either prevent these problems or help our body rebuild itself from prior damage done." I like to call these our lifestyle offsets and most times these are basic healthy habits that when done with consistency are powerful when it comes to most structural mobility issues and chronic disease.

Our health and that of our family will be a large Financial and Independence Asset in the future!

HYDRATION HELPS KEEP OUR CELLS YOUNG!

Hydration is next in line to oxygen in importance to sustain life! We have several trillion cells that get highly upset if they start to dry out! Its simple, keeping our cells hydrated helps keep them young, healthy and fighting disease!

Research in the field of cellular hydration has shown that when cells absorb water and swell (cellular hydration), this action acts as a positive stimulus. An increase in cellular hydration triggers the anabolic (rebuilding/recovery) mechanism and this anabolic state is then accompanied by a positive nitrogen balance, protein synthesis and growth hormone release.

Cellular hydration results in a balanced pH (makes our body less disease friendly), increased fat burning and reduced free radical damage (aging). When cells become dehydrated, this triggers a catabolic reaction or degenerative state, resulting in muscle wasting, inflammation and a greater risk of injury. Isn't it awesome that something we oft times take for granted may help in slowing the aging process and disease if done in adequate amounts with consistency?

Understanding how hydration of our cells work: Water moves in and out of the cells with electrolytes. Electrolytes are chemicals that form electrically charged ions (particles) in body fluids. I like to think of sodium and potassium as our entry and exit doors, and when kept in balance we keep a good flow going through the rooms/ partitions in our body that we call cells. These ions they form carry the electrical energy necessary for numerous physiological functions including muscle contractions and the transmission of nerve impulses, as well as many other bodily functions that are dependent on electrolytes.

Optimal performance requires a consistent and adequate supply of these electrolytes.

Did you know that when you sweat, you lower your fluid volume in your body thus lowering the amount of blood volume that your heart has to work with? This will then cause your heart to have to beat more rapidly to circulate your blood!

How to stay hydrated: Try to drink approximately half of your body weight in oz. of water everyday! Your best bet is staying consistent with your water intake along with an occasional sports drink (such as Gatorade or Powerade) and even better, a homemade natural electrolyte drink. If you sweat a lot, keeping an electrolyte drink within close range and convenience can really help save the day! However, drinking to many sports drinks when you're not sweating much can cause fluid retention. When you're very active or sweating a lot an occasional electrolyte drink should be adequate.

Take away: Hydration and staying active are about the cheapest but most effective forms of prevention of chronic disease that we have access to. We are made up of trillions of cells and if it only takes 3 days of no hydration for complete cellular death, can you imagine how many billion cells die in a half day with no hydration? Going a half day without hydrating will not cause us to die in whole, but it will certainly in part.

When we start not feeling well, one of the first questions we should ask ourselves is... could it simply be a lack of consistent hydration over the past 1-3 days?

HEART DISEASE, THE NUMBER ONE KILLER!

The way things stand now, one out of three people will die from a heart attack or cardiopulmonary related disease.

Heart Disease is the leading cause of death here in the United States and it hit my home area hard by the loss of 4 men, age range 46-50 in a one-week period in July of 2012. Heart disease is hereditary in my family and took my cousin Jimmy at only 23 years of age.

We have to look at what we are doing different, and the two largest changes seem to be, what we eat and our activity levels. We have also been advised to eat low fat foods, which is a complete farce. The problem with fat happens when we get a spike in sugar levels when consuming a high fat meal. They are finding now, that the real culprit to our cardiopulmonary system is sugar.

If we focus on some of the leading causes of heart disease and the lifestyle offsets for each one, it will help us counter this deadly disease. Chronic disease is very life and life style interruptive! A lifestyle offset simply works like a support for a weak or broken body part.

Culprits of Heart Disease: HYPERTENSION- HIGH CHOLESTEROL- OBESITY- DIABETES- STRESS- CIGARETTS

The first 5 are oft times preventable and treatable through diet, exercise, weight reduction and staying at a good weight and we all know how to lower the effects of cigarettes.

Tips:

If you feel your blood pressure rising: take a slow walk, or some slow continuous state exercise or activity. This will start warming your blood and works as a vasodilation (relaxation) of your blood vessels allowing for better blood flow thus lowering blood pressure.

If you have high cholesterol: Eat foods high in Omega 3 and heart healthy fats such as flaxseeds, soybeans, pumpkin seeds, pecans, tuna, salmon, mackerel and herring. Also start eating foods high in soluble fiber, such as legumes, seeds, nuts, beans, vegetables and fruits, eat these especially with high fat meals. Soluble fiber helps lower cholesterol by carrying out bile through our stool.

Note: your body produces bile to digest fats and the soluble fiber keeps it from absorbing back into your system so that you pass it out through your waste. This forces your body to make more bile and your liver makes new bile salts with guess what--- **cholesterol!**

Important: keep in mind that you are made up of cells and every cell in your body needs cholesterol for proper function, keeping cells from crystallizing, bile production for digestion, hormone production, helps nerves communicate with each other, combination of UV light from the sun and cholesterol in the skin helps make vitamin D. This list could continue, but I'm sure you get the point.

 Obesity: Exercise and stay active. Stay away from sugary foods and drink, also stay away from high calorie intake prior to periods of inactivity- as your body stores energy it doesn't need in your fat cells.

Diabetes: Most of the diabetes we hear about is Type 2 and most times is brought on by a sugary, starchy, high carbohydrates diet and lack of physical activity. Insulin spikes resulting from sugar spikes cause lesions and plaque in the arteries, this is responsible for hardening of the arteries and for cholesterol sticking to the arteries.

Stress: Try to stay stress free. Stress puts a load on the systems of our body that we're not meant to continue to carry and makes it so they cannot work properly, (whether mental or physical). If you're going through stressful times or situations, it's crucial that you find your de-stressing niche! Meditation techniques are helpful and whether a believer or not prayer has been proven to help. When you're stressed and worried, prayer combined with faith simply feels good when you can hand it over to Someone that you know can and wants to handle it. What works for someone else may not work for you, so find out what it is that can totally engage mind and body. Oft times when you come back to the situation, it will not have control over you, but you over it!

Cigarettes: If you smoke cigarettes, quit! If you buy cigarettes to smoke, you are paying and taking out time to hurt yourself by inhaling toxic chemicals that hurt the lining of your arteries. It also makes your lungs look like the inside of a smoke stack and you're putting in jeopardy the most important thing for life support, which is your capability for oxygen intake and uptake.

Medicine can be a very important part of intervening between us and chronic disease, but keeping medicine ahead of lifestyle changes for any chronic disease is like staying tethered to a tow truck after you're out of the ditch and the longer you stay tied to it the more counter productive the tow truck becomes, it simply doesn't work and this backwards way of doing things will eventually cause other problems. When you take medicine your body has to recover or deal with two things, and the longer you stay on the medicine, the more likely you will suffer from the potential side effects on the warning label.

Our heart beats around 100,000 times a day carrying blood and other nutrients to the rest of our body and when it stops we stop, so lets take care of that lil-fist sized thing!

CANCER, THE NUMBER TWO KILLER!

Though cancer comes in 2nd behind heart disease, it is probably the most dreaded diagnosis between the two. There are many categories of cancer but quite simply they are named after the part of the body where the cancer started even if it spreads to other parts of our body.

Please keep this in mind: Our body fights cancer EVERY day! It can simply be through a series of battles over a period of many years that our body no longer has the weaponry to fight it back into submission, and a doctor is able to diagnose what has accumulated as cancer. That is why it is so important that we keep a healthy immune system. The immune system works 24 hours a day, 7 days a week, 365 days a year as a shield to fight back cancer and other degenerative diseases. The 3 worse things we can do (when our body is hurting already) is use radiation which has been proven to increase cancer risk, chemotherapy which is a poisonous carcinogen, as well as surgeries and biopsies which can have an explosive like effect on spreading the cancer.

All cancers start in our cells. Our body produces trillions of cells each year to replace the prior generation; this is how we can start looking healthier and younger when we replace bad habits with healthy habits. These cells are supposed to grow in a very controlled manner and when we have abnormal cells that start growing in an out of control fashion it becomes what we call cancer. It works a little like rust does on metal if it's not stopped.

Lifestyle factors and genetics can be an issue when we look at whether or not we have an increased risk. Lifestyle factors can range from not only things we do to ourselves, but also the environmental exposures that we may know or not know about. When we inherit a gene that is linked to a certain cancer, it can increase our chances for that particular cancer. All of us fight cancer everyday, what is important is finding out what we can do, or discontinue to eliminate the aggravation that is causing the cancer, and then what we can do to heal this area back into sync with the rest of our body.

 What we can do: adapt lifestyle offsets for what is causing the cancer. Cancer is caused from a continued source of aggravation. If we can find and eliminate what is causing the aggravation, our body can begin shrinking and healing the cancer.

1. Take inventory and make sure there is nothing we are putting in our body that is undermining its capability to fight off cancer such as smoking and a diet filled with sugars and processed foods. Sugars are fuel to cancer, decreasing sugar and starch intake starves and shrinks cancer.

2. Look for things you can do that can build your immune system. Most times the things that build a healthy immune system are the healthy basic habits such as, staying hydrated, a diet rich in fruits and vegetables, stay active, work up a sweat regularly and get deep quality rest.

3. Lower meat intake and load up with enzymes, (especially the ones that help with digesting protein). Cancer shields itself from the immune system's capability to recognize it with a tough protein fibrin shield. When we have more free circulating enzymes in our blood, it helps eat away the protein shield, which in turn exposes the underlying cancer to our immune system, which then can kill the cancer.

4. If you have the potential of inheriting cancer through your genes, research, research, research, this is the way you will find the things in your life that you need to strengthen to help offset your genetic weakness.

If we can keep our immune system built up with the healthy basics it will do its best to fight the silent battles going on within us and will form a protective shield around us!

MEDICAL MISTAKES, NUMBER THREE KILLER

This article is to appeal to each and every one of us to take personal responsibility for our health and for the ones we care about. You have a lot more time to take personal responsibility for your health then your doctor or healthcare office does and you care a lot more then they do about your health and wellbeing.

To be fair, though medical errors is one of the top leading killers the medical field also saves a lot of lives through critical trauma and intervention.

Where we go wrong is being lead to believe that we need to constantly be tethered to the healthcare system through checkups, screenings, vaccinations and other regular office visits where we really don't know why we were there in the first place. The medical industry has wrongfully stepped into the shoes of prevention with what they call managed care. This is where they simply help you manage a disease, (curing nothing) and potentially cause a new side effect or chronic disease by the continued diagnostics, medicines or something you pick up from the medical practice or hospital.

We need to remember when we spend time in doctor's offices, clinics and hospitals, going through unnecessary procedures, the more time we spend in gathering places for sick people. We could spend that time trying to set up or reinforce healthy habits that will give our body the tools it needs to become and then stay healthy.

Our body's internal doctor (our immune system) is constantly going through a system of checks and balances, checking for errors, infections, muscle breakdown, bone density and many other system checks and it comes back with a report of the list of things needed. Often this is a very simple list of needs, clean oxygen, staying hydrated, a more balanced diet, regular exercise, de-stressing regularly and getting good deep rest.

Our body has a similar reaction to our car when we let the fluids get out of whack, or when we put in fluids that it doesn't like or recognize, it will simply not run properly and if we don't start using the right fluids, something a lot worse will happen such as engine or transmission failure.

We are heading into an era where the healthcare system is going to have a lot more new people entering due to the aging baby-boom population, so for us to believe the fallacies in the healthcare system will improve as they try to handle a lot more patients is putting ourselves at risk.

One offset that we have that can help us counter limited access healthcare is our easy access to information and the internet to research whatever health issue you may be facing. As many of us as possible should try to learn how to use the internet for health research, it is a powerful diagnostic tool and unlike your doctor it will allow you unlimited amounts of time for free to ask health and medical questions.

Doing your own diagnostics: I want to share how I research something on the Internet. I like using information from the Lance Armstrong website "for health related research, so if I want to research what the best foods are for a diabetic or borderline diabetic, I'll go to the search bar and type in what I'm researching with "livestrong" at the end of my question.

Example: For foods that are best for a diabetic, I'll type the following into the search bar, "best foods for a diabetic livestrong," then I'll click on the link that looks the most informative for what I'm researching, and continue narrowing my research from there. You can also watch videos on your health topic by entering YouTube at the end of your question.

Example: Diabetes YouTube. Pick videos that have a large number of views (this shows that it's probably a credible source that has a large following).

Try this: Think of something (anything) that you may want to know more about, then go on the internet and research it for one hour and see how much you can learn in one hour for free!

If we can take personal responsibility for our own health and the ones around us by implementing healthy habits that our bodies can depend on and learn to use the power of the internet to research health, prevention and medicine, I believe we will have some of the best sets of tools we can add to our arsenal to help us offset an uncertain healthcare system.

Take away: If we can get proactive in learning what helps our body stay healthy now, we greatly increase our chance of not being reliant on the healthcare system later!

DIABETES, THE SLEEPING GIANT AMONG US!

Diabetes is actually the 3rd on the list of death by chronic disease, but is 4th behind medical misdiagnosis and hospital infections and is the number one cause of amputations!

It is not an easy task to research exactly why or how a person gets diabetes and this is in part due to so many different gene and lifestyle factors that we face as individuals. So instead of focusing on how we get diabetes, I would rather focus on what we can do to help us better deal with or possibly prevent this dreaded disease and decrease our reliance on medical intervention to counter diabetes by using every lifestyle offset that we can, to minimize the effect it has on our life and the ones we care about.

First we need to look at how our diets have changed. We eat a lot more packaged and processed foods (that are either artificially sweetened or breakdown rapidly into sugar) then we used to, and a lot of these foods cause a sharp spike in blood sugar.

Example of why: processed food and drinks such as candies, deserts, sodas, sweat tea, fruit drinks, etc. do not have the soluble fiber that comes with nature's sweets. These fruits have their own soluble fiber that slows the absorption (of the sugars they contain) into our system, (God knew what he was doing when he designed nature's sweets)!

A high carbohydrate, starchy diet will constantly keep our blood sugar spiked from the rapid breakdown of these foods into sugar, and this will continue to place a demand on the pancreas to produce more insulin. Insulin is the hormone that helps unlock the cells of our body to transport energy and nutrients into them, when this need is satisfied it will take the left over energy and put it into our liver and fat cells for later use.

Second we need to look at how activity burns off extra blood sugars. Insulin needs to take the extra glucose somewhere, either to muscles that need the energy or to the liver for our backup supply and after this it has no choice but to store it in our fat cells, (this is what makes them larger and is simply our insulin working properly). If this process does not happen and our insulin cannot regulate and remove the excess sugars from our blood it can cause a sticky gooey mess in our system that can start to cause things like blindness, and poor circulation that can lead to amputations of our extremities. So it's really important that our insulin is able to regulate the levels of glucose in the blood.

Two things can happen when you constantly put an overload of sugar into your bloodstream;

1. The cells that make up our body start to get resistant to a constant barrage of insulin and will become less responsive, and when this happens it forces the pancreas to produce a stronger surge of insulin to overcome the resistance the cells are putting up.

2. Your pancreas which produces the insulin may get wore out and fatigued and start producing less and less insulin causing you to become insulin dependent on an outside source.

Take away:

Diet: When we eat something that is high in carbohydrates, such as casseroles, spaghetti, and other starchy foods, avoid desserts or sugary drinks! It is easy to add in an extra 100 grams of sugar, simply by what we choose to drink or by adding a dessert! Eat foods that absorb into your system slower. Add foods that are rich in soluble fiber to your meals (to slow the absorption of sugars into your blood) such as- legumes, seeds, nuts, beans and lentils. You can also keep a bottle of BeneFiber (or other) soluble fiber powder around to mix in or sprinkle over your foods. A good way to see if its soluble or insoluble fiber is, soluble fiber mixes easily in water and insoluble fiber clumps up. Insoluble fiber helps push food through your system and helps with waste elimination, and soluble fiber forms a gel like substance in your digestive track that helps slow down sugar's entry into your blood.

If we could get a good picture of the pain and misery that sugar loaded foods too often can cause in our lives, they probably wouldn't look and taste so good!

Food tip: When you know you are entering a period of very little activity or inactivity, really slow down on the foods high in carbohydrates and sugars. These are fast fuel foods and can cause problems when too much is consumed during periods of low energy output. If these foods are the only ones available, cut way back on the portions as your body doesn't feel the calorie overload until about 15 minutes later due to a lack of insoluble fiber in most of these foods.

Exercise and staying active: Exercise and staying active helps your body burn off extra blood sugars that your body has to otherwise figure out what to do with and also keeps your cells more insulin sensitive.

Exercise tip: Do a full body exercise, such as rapid squatting and standing arms thrusting upward for about 1-3 minutes, 5 minutes prior to eating and 1 hour after eating, this helps make your muscle cells more receptive to the glucose from the meal, takes a burden off of the pancreas and helps guard us against insulin resistance.

Lets keep this sleeping giant (diabetes), in a sleep-induced coma through our healthy lifestyle choices starting today!

OBESITY...THE COMMON LINK TO MOST CHRONIC DISEASE

When we look at statistics and see how much of the population is overweight the numbers are staggering and obesity's link to most chronic disease is really scary!

Diet and lack of adequate activity are the two main contributing factors to this epidemic, so if we can start making some very simple lifestyle changes we not only can change our physical shape, we can also increase our body's capability to fight illness and disease.

The fight against obesity is one that is particularly interesting to me since it's the business I've been in since 1991 and probably the main reason that most people want to start exercising and dieting. I have seen many fad diets, pills and dietary shakes come and go and after all these, common sense prevails and is the one that comes out on top every time. If we can get a good clear image in our mind of the root causes of obesity, we can get into the shape we want, without spending our money to lose weight. Isn't it ironic how much money we as Americans spend on consuming more food then we should and are one of the only countries in the world that will turn around and pay for diet pills, shakes etc., to lose the fat our body stored from the extra food consumed.

There are a few things I have categorized below that are prime culprits in causing the obesity epidemic...

First: If we look at what has changed in our diets and lifestyles in general we can find the reason this is an ongoing battle for us or for the ones around us that we care about.

Example: A boy or girl is very active throughout high school through various activities and sports, he or she is consuming enough calories to sustain this activity and body weight and growth, but then after school this graduate takes an office job and continues to eat about the same amount of food, these extra unburned calories turn to fat. If a person gets inactive and their caloric burn rate is 500 calories less per day then before, this adds up! 500 calories x 30 days =15,000 calories and there is only 3,500 calories in a pound of fat, this can really add up in a year's time!

Second: Inactivity causes our muscles to lose their tone and muscles losing their tone are like turning the heat down on a stove it slows the muscles capability to burn calories. A loss in metabolism has more to do with a loss in muscle tone then it has to do with getting older.

Exercise all parts of the body so that both upper and lower body muscles as well as core muscles can do their fair share in boosting your metabolism.

Third: Our diets are so loaded with calorie dense foods that have little or no fiber in them and this makes so that we cannot feel that we overate until its too late. Small amounts of food that have a lot of calories in only a few bites (calorie dense foods) can be great for when we don't have time to eat, but only in small amounts. Deserts and sweet drinks can easily add an extra 300-500 extra calories on top of a meal that was already adequate.

Releasing fat: In order to release stored fat to be used as burnable energy, we need to keep our intake of sugary and starchy foods to a minimum. Sugar has been THE BAD culprit for a lot of the obesity epidemic and if I would have a choice of the two worst words in lending to the problem and making people feel good about eating foods that were not good for them, it would be the food label Fat Free.

Insulin produced as a result of sugar in the blood will lock up the release mechanisms on your fat cells. When lowering your sugar, starches and carbohydrates for one to two days it can be beneficial for weight loss to have a cheat meal, this is for the purpose of refueling your muscle cells. If you don't refuel in time, your body will think it is starving so it breaks down muscle for energy so as to slow your metabolism down and accommodate the new low calorie schedule. If you go really low on the calorie intake, don't do it for longer then 2 days before you have a cheat day, however keep sugary food and drink to a minimum or you'll erase your weight loss efforts.

Take away: You do not have to spend money to lose weight! The best way is to make some simple lifestyle changes, take in fewer calories, burn some extra calories through adding in exercise, drink half your body weight in ounces of water, and every few days (after your low calorie days) have a good cheat meal to replenish the energy in your muscle cells.

Lets keep our body from toting more weight then it was designed to carry, it will feel better, look better and help us fight chronic diseases!

YOUR BODY "YOUR UNIVERSAL GYM"

We get bombarded throughout the year with ads promoting super supplements, weight loss pills, weight loss plans, and exercise machines, so its no wonder that it has a psychological effect on what we feel is necessary for health and fitness. Though some of these work really well, the problem is when these ads make someone feel they "have to have it" for increasing their level of fitness.

What each of us needs to know is that we have enough body weight to give us the resistance we need to get a good exercise routine wherever we're at, whenever we want and the only cost is your time. When we move our body weight at a faster pace it increases the resistance and done consistently over a period of time these muscles used for the movement will build and develop to accommodate the new stress, (this is the strengthening and toning process in a nutshell).

When you use functional exercise movements (that you use in everyday living) for your exercise, you strengthen and condition this part of your life. When we do something like stooping or squatting to pick something up we would really be surprised if we could see the muscular mechanics going to work to make this movement possible. When we repeat this same movement several times at a faster speed or add extra resistance or weight, we strengthen the muscles, bones, tendons and ligaments used to do this and it becomes easier!

Example: Many times when a person falls, its the first time in a long time that they were actually laid out on the floor, and now the person is possibly hurt and is faced with having to get back up from a position they are not used to being in. If a person would get down on the floor and then get back up several times, (slowly at first) and gradually pick up the pace, it could give someone a pretty good workout. When we mimic the movements we use in real life (in our exercise routine) it makes our activities of daily living (ADL's) easier and whether an young athlete or a senior, it simply helps us handle our day better.

 Take away: Find an exercise or 2 that gets most of your skeletal muscles moving, (such as a squat thrust). Do this by squatting and then rising to the front of your foot with arms thrusting upward. Do the movement slowly and don't squat too deep. As you get used to this, do a deeper squat and speed up the movement. The 3 main things you want to work toward are:

1. Range of motion.

2. Speed of movement.

3. Length of time that you can go before resting.

A good short workout to intensify the above would be to go from the squat thrust exercise and then lay down on the floor and do pushups, (beginners can keep the knees against the floor to decrease resistance). The speed of movement in most any exercise you do increases the resistance and it results in increased muscle strength, size and bone density. So whether confined to your office, home or on the road, you carry your gym with you wherever you go if you have a few basic movements that activate the large muscle groups of the body! Try getting down flat on the floor, stomach or back and get back up lifting your arms above your head and see how many times you can do this, it's like a full body power jog!

Full body movements done with intensity = Results! The key to getting results and at the same time preventing injury is gradually increasing the range of motion, speed, and length of time doing the exercises.

Remember: steady wins the race!

OUR WHITE FOOD COCAINES "SALT AND SUGAR"

Neurological studies have shown very similar activity in the brain with salt and sugar as with cocaine. Hmm guess it doesn't take a rocket scientist to understand why foods loaded with sugar and salt have so much value to the food industry!

With the massive surge in obesity, diabetes and heart disease, it's sheer craziness if we do not draw a straight line between what we consume and inactivity. Processed sugars, salts, sodium nitrates and aspartame (artificial sweeteners) are all major changes in the western diet, so we should be looking at these as something that may be feeding the problems of obesity, diabetes, and heart disease.

Note: this chapter is to address the over usage of refined sugars and salts, not sugar and salt in its raw natural state. Also if you cook and prepare your food from scratch, there are a lot of health benefits from adding in some natural salt. Most people however get too much in the typical western diet and most of it is refined.

 Salt: salt helps your body to retain fluid, some is good but a continuous over consumption can create too much volume in your blood causing a higher blood pressure. Over consumption of salty foods (without its potassium counter partner) can cause water retention and this done long enough will distort our shape!

 Sugar: sugar in our drinks and candies (without soluble fiber like fruits have) can absorb too rapidly into the bloodstream causing a spike in blood sugar. This in turn causes a big burst of insulin from your pancreas to help transport sugars to cells throughout the body, (vital tissues first, fat cells second). This done over a long enough period of time (since fat cells store our extra calories) will distort our shape as well.

  At the same time the sugar and salt content in the foods and drinks we consume has gone up, our activity levels have dropped. We eliminate a lot of salt through sweating as well as burn off the extra sugars by staying active and when we do not do this it simply allows these things to build up in our body in the form of water retention and stored body fat.

When we truly connect the chronic diseases that are linked to excessive weight in our minds and how most of it is connected to our choice in consumption, it can really help us in our food and drink choices.

Whether its an eventual heart attack or stroke that makes so we can no longer perform like we used to, or diabetes (which can cause circulatory problems that in turn brings on awful things such as amputations and blindness), these carbonated, caffeinated, sugar and salt loaded food and drink products will probably not look so good to us!

It takes 90-120 days for our blood supply to be replaced by a new blood supply; it takes around 6 months for our soft tissue to be replaced and around -12 months for a complete cellular regeneration, all the way to our bone and tooth enamel! The above is made up from the food choices, drink choices, as well as the environment we have been exposed to during this time period! Keep in mind that new cell generations are mutations from the prior generation of cells, so restoring complete vibrancy and health on a cellular level does not happen overnight. A healthy and active lifestyle done with consistency is key to maintaining or returning to good health.

We not only are what we eat but we also become what we do with what we eat!

HOW TO BUILD MUSCLE AND HOW BUILDING MUSCLE BUILDS BONE DENSITY

We build and strengthen muscle FIRST by a breaking down process through the introduction of a new stressor that our body is not familiar with.

Our body's natural response to a new stressor is to compensate by strengthening that area simply so it doesn't get so stressed out the next time it has to repeat the same action. If we repeat the same activity, we simply maintain that level of fitness, BUT if we increase the intensity, it forces the muscles to adapt to a new level of strength.

Atrophy: when we decrease these activities or stressors our body senses less need for strength in that area and will atrophy (shrink) strength in that area. This is pretty much the same whether in mental or physical exercise. As we age we tend to get more inactive due to less responsibilities, so as a natural response our body shrinks unnecessary muscle mass and bone density. The first biomarker that indicates the beginning signs of the aging process is a decrease in protein (muscle) in the body and the two largest contributing factors to this is inactivity and diet.

It is pretty simple to take steps to avoid this if we keep up the level and variety of activities throughout our life. A lot of times after long periods of inactivity, we suddenly put exercise or the same level of activity back on the body and wind up getting injured as a result and then blame it on aging. It's not so much that we're older, its all the inactivity that has caused us to lose strength in our muscles, tendons and ligaments, which at the same time leads to loss in bone density.

The scale can give us a false sense of security if we become inactive and simply try to keep the scale weight the same. When we become inactive, we should drop in weight due to the loss in muscle tone and bone density since these are large contributing factors to our overall body mass.

As our body becomes more fatty, and our muscles, tendons, ligaments and bones lose their strength, our weight begins to hang more heavily on them causing rapid aging to our skeletal structure. This can also give us a false sense of aging (due to achy muscles, bones, and joints) however inactivity is the culprit, NOT aging.

The way we build muscle: (this includes seniors) is to break down muscle fibers first simply by demanding more from them then they are used to. Your body will naturally build them back stronger in case this stress happens again. So when you want to strengthen muscles all over your body, you need more then just walking, jogging, you need exercises that include the pulling and pushing muscles of the upper body as in functional everyday movements!

Example: Squatting and picking up an object such as a gallon jug and then lifting it above your head, (repeat this action for a few repetitions) and over time increase the resistance by speeding up the movement.

How building muscle builds bone density:

The tugging action of active muscles pulling the skeletal structure through a variety of movements will signal the brain for an increase in bone mass to counter the new demands we are placing on it. When we do a variety of exercises to strengthen muscles all over our body it also stimulates bone density over our entire body.

  Since the first signs of the aging process starting is loss of muscle mass, we can slow the effects of aging by stimulating muscle growth no matter what our age!

 If we don't use muscle we lose it, so lets use it, retain it and gain it!!!

HOW DOES PROTEIN BUILD NEW MUSCLE?

After we make a muscle or group of muscles work harder then they are used to, small micro fibers in our muscles break. If overdone or overtrained, our muscles can become too broken down and in this state of disrepair could lead to injury if we do not give it adequate recovery time before doing the same exercises or activities again. When these muscles are not fully recovered, they are also weaker thus putting more pressure on tendons and ligaments when you train to soon again because of the surrounding muscle not being as supportive.

There are 3 things that help strengthen, tone and build muscle: 1st a breaking down of muscle tissue, 2nd a balanced diet, 3rd deep rest and recovery.

Our focus today is on how protein in our diet
builds new muscle or helps recondition and tone old muscle. Our muscle is made up of protein, but when worked hard can break down small muscle fibers into amino acids that we can burn as energy. Pretty much the reverse of this happens when we eat protein. Our dietary protein breaks down into amino acids, that your body will absorb and use to rebuild broken down muscle/ protein which is in effect building new muscle that is built back stronger then it was before.

I like to think of the proteins that we eat as being
a process where our body takes the protein and converts it into amino acid patch paint to make muscular repairs throughout the body. Once this amino patch paint adheres onto the broken down muscle, it becomes new muscle helping us to create a younger muscle environment that is toned and stronger.

One of my favorite sources of protein is the egg.

Other good sources of protein come from a variety of meats, (fish, chicken, occasional red meat) and

dairy along with cholesterol lowering protein foods such as beans, lentils, nuts and seeds. With protein being the building block for new muscle, we need to make sure the protein we eat is quality material!

New muscle means younger muscle and the

action of toning this muscle helps strengthen bones while at the same time shaping the body, toning the body, and bringing back mobility as we get older that we thought was a disappearing act...

Isn't it awesome that we can do a remodeling of our body, health and mobility no matter what our age?

FAT CELLS ARE OUR MICRO FUEL TANKS

We have billions of these little fuel cells, and though fat gets a bad rap because most of us would like less of it, it actually serves a very vital energy role in the body. When we lose body fat we are not referring to the cell but rather the energy matter inside the cell. These cells are like micro balloons that can expand as needed (to accommodate the excess calories we eat) and shrink as we expend the energy. The only way to remove fat cells is surgically, but we can however shrink them if we're trying to lose weight.

We have fat cells all over our body for the purpose of reserve fuel for when our energy level runs low in our main fuel tank, which is our stomach, intestines, bloodstream and liver. When we constantly keep enough calories in our main fuel tank for our daily activities, we don't store any excess, but we don't burn off any of our stored energy either. When we know that we ate too much, it can be very beneficial to skip the next meal and burn off some of this excess fuel before we eat again!

Example: If I know that I ate too much for dinner, I'll simply skip eating until around 1 pm the next day to burn off those extra calories.

When we take in more fuel then we will burn between the times that we eat, we simply store the extra. If we continue to do this long enough those billions of little fat cells will continue to expand and make us look fat. The exact opposite happens when we regularly use up the energy in our fat cells causing them to shrink. The problem many of us have is getting these fat cells to release their energy.

Here are 2 ways we can open up this reserve energy source:

1. We can: increase our heart rate by about 50-70% (depending on physical condition) for at least a steady 20 minutes or more. This will trigger what most of us know as our 2nd wind, it's actually our body starting to burn body fat. Our body is designed to detect a need for energy, when our heart rate is increased for a sustained period, thus signaling the need for a strong source of energy to sustain the activity. I like to think of it as starting a fire... 1st comes the kindling and when that builds up enough fire and heat, the logs will catch on fire and that's when the real heat and energy starts!

2. We can: drop the amount of calories to a very low level for an extended period, forcing our body to tap into reserve fuel thus dropping the level of energy matter in our fat cells. If we do this for too long however, our body will think its starving and will recognize the need to slow down our metabolism, it will do this by burning muscle tissue instead of fat because it is the most metabolically active. You can avoid this by not doing more then 2 super low calorie days in a row, or no more then 18-24 hours complete fast.

Remember: staying low calorie all the time will simply force our body into accommodating this by burning off some muscle, and when this happens our metabolism slows down so that you can survive on this starvation diet.

Our body shifts between energy from sugars, carbohydrates and fats. A sugar load entering, (or constantly supplying) the blood with glucose from sugary or starchy foods, will lock up your fat cells until the insulin level (from the intake of sugars) drops back down.

We have been blessed with a body that can shift all kinds of gears to accommodate our energy needs, and the simple basics of refueling our body, and fuel depletion work today just like it did thousands of years ago!

WHY IS MY METABOLISM SLOWING DOWN?

This is not tied with aging nearly so much as it is with a gradual loss of muscle and muscle tone as we get older. Even if we keep our weight the same, as we become less active our muscles lose their tone and more of our weight is coming from a gradual gain of fat. When our muscles lose their strength, density and tone its like turning our burners on low heat, our body simply does not burn calories like it used to.

Most of us (after the age of 35) lose enough muscle every year to burn 4 pounds of fat! This means that we're not only losing the only thing on our body that creates strength, tone and good shape, we also are losing the very thing that helps us keep our metabolism up. So just like the simplicity of turning up the burners on our stove to generate more heat, we can also turn up our capability of burning fat and calories by toning and building muscle.

Toned muscle weighs more then un-toned muscle, so it's very easy for an average height person to gain 8-12 pounds of weight in the muscle sector, (when starting a fitness routine). This is why the weight doesn't drop nearly as rapidly on the scale the first few months.

Example: if we gain 10 lb. of muscle and lose 10 lb. of fat, the scale weight hasn't changed, but our shape sure has! Since this new muscle adds to the thermogenic heat in your body your metabolism is changing as well. The same principle applies, that we should drop body weight if we get inactive to compensate for weight loss from muscle tone. If we continue to weigh the same, we can count on it that we gained body fat, (this is why our shape looks so different, even though our weight stays the same on the scale).

To help insure that we're properly turning on our thermogenic heat to its full potential, we need to exercise the muscles all over our body. We can do this by making sure that our exercise routine includes, pulling, pushing and pressing, (these each get different muscle groups).

Example: rowing gets the back and biceps, pushups get our triceps and chest, leg press, squats with weights or body weight squats get most of the large muscle groups of the legs. Keep a basic routine, but try to add some different angles to your pulling, pushing and pressing movements to give the muscle groups better development.

Example home routine: after walking or some other form of warm-up, lay on the floor and do pushups until tiring, then get up and pick up a weighted object off the floor and straighten to standing position, repeat this action until tiring and then do some squats with arms extended out in front of you, raising your arms toward ceiling as you come to a standing position. Repeat this circuit about 3 times and then finish routine by getting on the floor and doing some crunches for stomach.

Remember: if toning muscle turns up our metabolism, shouldn't we tone muscle all over our body?

Take away: turning up our own metabolism by toning our muscles is the cheapest form of a weight loss program and it is also THE healthiest way!

THE THERMIC EFFECT OF FOOD

Most of us really like when our body has a high rate of thermogenesis (burning fat for energy), but did you know that not only can toned muscle burn more calories, the foods we choose to eat can also make a difference as well! Some foods make the body work harder (to break them down into usable fuel and nutrients that our body can absorb), then others do, and in doing so causes us to burn more calories throughout the digestive period, this is "The Thermic Effect of Food."

Example: when we intake a good source of protein, up to 30% of the calories in the protein can be burned just for digestion purposes.

The foods that would be on the lower end of the thermic burn chart would be sugary foods, starchy foods and foods with very little fiber. These foods absorb very rapidly into our bloodstream and besides using very little calories to digest them, they can also cause very rapid spikes in blood sugars. These foods can be good fuel when ate in low amounts prior to periods of intense activity. This is because of us needing a fuel that our body doesn't have to work hard to breakdown and since we need our blood going to our working muscles instead of our digestive track, this can be a good time to eat some fast absorbing foods.

Remember: the key is in eating low quantities of fast burning fuel. These foods are the ones that have a lot of calories in even small amounts of food and it's easy to over consume since they don't have much fiber and it's not till later that we feel the effects of all these extra calories.

I think its pretty neat when you look at an experienced cook's meal and can see the different fuels/foods on the plate and as long as we watch our portion sizes, we usually can have different stages of fuel from the meal that will sustain us for hours!

When we get to know what amount of energy output we have coming up, it can be a guide as to which foods we should eat more of.

Example: if we know we're going to be setting at the desk for the rest of the day, with little activity, we should go really light on the starches, simple carbohydrates, sweet foods and drinks. But if we know that we are really going to have a lot of energy output for the next hour, we could eat some of the above in small amounts and it would be great short-term energy. Just remember, this can fuel the body for the short run, but in general it's much better to eat a balanced meal where the starches, simple carbohydrates, sweet food and drink are very much kept in moderation.

For a learning exercise do Internet searches on: The thermic effect of food.

Take away: Rapid absorbing fuel if ate in excess before periods of low or no activity will be stored for later use in our fat cells and this is what makes them balloon in size.

If we pretend we're a car and that we **are** going on

a leisure road trip or are setting still idling, lets not

use the same type of fuel as a racecar does in a 1/4-

mile stretch!

ECONOMY OF MOVEMENT

Most of us know what it means to be in a tough economic environment whether it was self imposed damage to our finances or outside circumstances that we did not have control over. Either way we know that it restricts what we're able to do, by limiting the flexible spending power we have, and it becomes really hard to do the same things we either used to do or want to do.

Economy of movement is much the same; we many times take it for granted, until we lose capability of movement for doing things like we used too and it takes much more effort to do the same thing and in some cases we are simply unable to do it at all. Unless through an accident or a debilitating disease, most times this loss of movement comes on us like a slow creep rust over time, that we recognize only when we try to do something that we haven't done in a long time. We then oft times take the most damaging approach and blame it on aging instead of the real culprit, inactivity!

When it takes an extreme amount of effort to do activities of daily living, (ADL) this is simply a bad economy of movement, but when we can do these same activities of daily living (ADL's) with ease, it means that we have a good economy of movement. And it will show in the ease in which we're able to handle our day whatever it may be!

Whether we're 25 years old or 85 years young this can really become important when (the very thing of walking across the floor to the door or playing in the yard with our children) becomes something that takes an extreme amount of effort. Once it gets to this point many of us avoid doing these things for the above same reason, and the problem usually then gets worse and gains more debilitating control of our life.

A vehicle will rust and corrode if it sets up too long, simply because the parts and fluids that were meant to move didn't, and we can expect anything from leaking gaskets, flat tires, rusting and other things that we could have prevented by regular usage and maintenance. Our body is much the same, if we don't move, activate and challenge the different parts of our body, a thing called sarcopenia shrinkage of muscle tissue will set in, and our body will begin to age much more rapidly.

There are several things we can do to avoid this:

1. We can replace discontinued activities with new ones.

Example: if we retire from active work, or are simply no longer the one doing the physical end of a job and start to manage it instead, such as spending a lot of our time behind a desk, we can then replace the physical work with exercise or active sports. We need to remember that when we are active, more of our weight is muscle and when we start to become inactive, we should lose weight due to a loss in muscle weight. Oft times (when we become inactive) we stay the same weight or gain weight, and the muscles, tendons, ligaments and bones become less supportive and movement becomes more and more labored.

2. Make sure that all parts of the body get exercised several times a week, whether individually or doing a functional movement/exercise (one used in natural movement) such as squatting and touching the floor and then reaching toward the ceiling (repeat movement as many times as you can). You can increase the resistance over time by speeding up your movement, or holding weights in your hand while doing the movement.

Take away: consistency wins this race, overdoing it is what usually leads to injury and can give us the false sense of aging, when it was simply too much activation after too long inactivation!

 Consistent physical activity does a lot to stimulate the physiological processes in our body that help guard us against premature aging, disease, and losing strength and capability to do our daily activities...

A body that keeps in motion stays in motion!

THE OBESITY CYCLE

We have put ourselves on a generational spinning wheel that is going to be catastrophic in the creation of a debt cycle (chronic disease) that we ARE GOING TO HAVE TO PAY if we don't change!

When we look back and factor in some things that have caused changes in our sizes and the changeover from infectious disease as a leading killer of Americans to now being chronic diseases- we can actually trace some of the main contributing factors very easily. During the years of the baby boomer's birth and growth years an abundance of fast food restaurants, processed foods, ever expanding sugared drink, candy and wheat products were made available. Many of these foods convert to energy very rapidly due to the starch or the sugar content, and when combined with high fat foods, can cause our body to store it if we are not very active in the following several hours. It so happens however that (as these products have become more and more available and considered as a regular food source), our activity levels have also slowed down, creating a perfect storm of obesity!

We have a food supply chain that has placed importance on bringing to market foods that can be grown in massive quantities to supply the demand of people who no longer grow their own food. So whether its meat product that is loaded with hormones and dripping with fat, combined with meals and snacks that is mostly made up of wheat and other starchy products, combined with a huge decrease in activity levels and energy expenditure, its no wonder that our size as a nation has increased so much!

These same products oft times don't have much insoluble fiber in them, so our I'm full signal doesn't give its signal in time, and we have that overstuffed feeling about 15 minutes later when its too late and way too much sugar and fats are entering our bloodstream. Our body simply compensates by flooding our system with insulin to start removing these excess calories from the blood and storing them for later use in our fat cells and, this is what makes us look fat!

Solutions:

1. We can do a kitchen cleanup of what we have so readily available to eat all around us and replace them with things like nuts, nut butters, berries, beans, vegetables some fruit, and other one ingredient foods. We can drink 1/2 our body weight in ounces of water. We can try to eat less bread and other wheat products such as crackers, and other pastries made with flour.

Example: if we're going to eat a hamburger, or hotdog, eat it with beans, vegetables and water to drink instead of bread, buns, chips and sodas or sweet tea.

2. Increase activity levels with things like walking, active sports/hobbies, and exercises that activate the pushing, pulling and pressing muscles of the body. There are also many ways to wiggle in a little physical exertion in our regular daily routine and if we can identify these activities of daily living (ADL's) and then do them with speed and can very easily burn an extra 500 calories a day by doing so!

1 pound of fat = 3500 calories

 We as a person, family, community, town and county can turn this around if we can figure out ways to keep ourselves inspired first. We can then inspire the ones we care about and the many others we come in contact with.

 We are not an island, our actions and habits have a ripple effect on the ones around us whether they're bad or good habits!

ALKALINE VS. ACIDIC = HEALTH VS. DISEASE

Simply put, an alkaline body is not disease friendly and the bad stuff has a hard time staying or growing, but an acidic environment does the opposite and if you keep your body alkaline instead of acidic, it can help you prevent disease!

Stress and diet are probably the main culprits in either creating an acidic build up or placing an acid load on the body. Stress can have this effect in part to shallow breathing caused by a tense stressed body and system, and when we take shallow breaths, we do not expel the carbon dioxide like we should. Our body is designed to break down this extra carbon dioxide build up and it will, but when we eat something like a cheese burger, fries and soda it will be busy trying to focus on the acid content in your digestive track, thus shelving the other environmental cleanup it has to do in our body until later. When we don't give ourselves a break, whether to de-stress or to eat foods that help balance out the more acidic ones, our body will become more and more acidic, thus becoming fertile breeding ground for diseases to start and grow!

Our body's backup plan if there are not enough alkalizing minerals in our diet (such as from fruits and vegetables) will release calcium, magnesium and potassium in the blood to buffer the acid. Our body will release stored minerals from our bones to buffer the acid if we do not have enough foods in our diet that provide this. This can cause a weakening of our bones.

Some of the most acidic items in our diet are: fish, meat, poultry, beans, sugar, starches, dairy, caffeine, alcohol and salt. However just because they are the more acidic foods does not at all mean they're all bad. It's when we don't counter the acid load with alkaline foods that things get out of balance. We can get the benefit of these foods but offset the acid load by adding in more fruits and vegetables with whatever we eat, it sort of works like a good marriage where one provides what the other cannot and vice versa, and in doing so, balance each other out causing good things to happen!

Good foods to add in to help offset the acid are: most fruits, (except cranberries), green leafy vegetables, broccoli, carrots, cauliflower, celery, onions, cottage cheese, flax seed and sprouts.

Try this: instead of just eating a turkey sandwich (which is a starch and meat) add in some raw broccoli and carrot sticks to eat as you're eating your sandwich.

Supplementation: there are a variety of fruit and vegetable drink powders and capsules that are available (in most nutrition stores) to help supplement meals that don't include fruits and vegetables. These fruit and vegetable concentrates are also a very good source of the antioxidants that help slow the aging process of our organs and bodies.

Relaxation: try to relax at least once a day even if for 10 minutes. Try to take in deep breaths and then slowly expel as much as you can, (this will help push old stale carbon dioxide out) and will also help lower stress levels.

Did you know that dirt could be either acidic or alkaline as well? The proper pH balance works the same way, if the dirt is too acidic only bad stuff will grow, but when in proper balance good things can grow! The earth and our body were both designed with awesome healing capabilities, but it's up to us to keep things in balance!

A HEALTHY IMMUNE SYSTEM = YOUR HEALTHCARE VACCINATION

A healthy immune system is definitely our best personal defense against an uncertain healthcare system and to help vaccinate us against the disease of healthcare system reliance!

Whenever we head into the fall season, we also head into the flu season and there are no shortages of advertisements warning us to get the flu vaccinations. What I would really like seeing more of is education on the value of building our own immune system through some healthy steps that do not suggest going to the medicine cabinet, drug store, doctor's offices, buying supplements and depending on a constant string of vaccinations. The pharmaceutical industry knows it has several hundred million potential customers in America alone that they can profit from by medicating us even when we're not sick, in other words, non-sick care.

Please don't get me wrong, vaccinations have their place, but we have headed down a path of dependency that is risky and even the medical profession knows they are operating in a grey area on. We have somehow left from primarily relying on the healthcare system for intervention to a reliance on them for prevention, which is not their specialty.

We have personalized designer vaccinations, which are our naturalized surroundings. If a person lives their life inside a sterilized bubble, in just a short time his or her immune system would greatly weaken.

Several weeks ago I wrote an article on how our muscle grows or gets stronger, by first breaking down. This simply happens when a muscle gets stressed more then it is used to, because of the heavier weight lifted or more repetitions being squeezed out. This causes breaking down of muscle fibers, and thus issues a signal from that area, not to only rebuild the broken down muscle fibers, but to build them back a little stronger so that it can handle the same stress load better the next time it happens. Our immune system works in much the same way, by using our surroundings combined with healthy habits to build a strong immune system. Here are some very important habits to build and maintain your immune system...

1. Stay active.

2. Balanced diet.

3. Stay hydrated.

4. Get plenty of deep rest.

Winter Tip: we get a lot less sun in the winter, which means we get a lot less vitamin D. This also happens to be when our immune system seems to suffer the most, could it possibly be connected to less vitamin D in our system??? So lets get out in the sun whenever we can during the winter, and if you take a vitamin D supplement, take it when you have eaten some food with fat in it since vitamin D is a fat-soluble vitamin.

Immune system tip: Drink some warm water with lemon before bed and when you wake up, (lemons are high in vitamin C and potassium). Vitamin C is great for fighting colds and potassium stimulates brain & nerve function and helps control blood pressure. Lemons also help balance our pH: believe it or not lemons are a very alkaline food. They are acidic on their own, but inside our bodies they're alkaline (the citric acid does not create acidity in the body once metabolized).

Remember: a slightly alkaline body is the key to good health and disease prevention!

 Healthy habits and your natural surroundings work together like a well-orchestrated symphony in their capability to protect and immunize you, God wasn't playing around when He designed your immune system!

HOW COLD WEATHER CAN REV YOUR METABOLISM!

We can usually feel our appetite go up in the winter, when we're exposed to the cold, (this is because our body is burning more fuel for heat)! Our normal resting body temperature should be at or around 97.6 degrees, so if its 30 degrees outside, our body has to fire up it's heaters!

 We have something called our BMR (Basal Metabolic Rate), which is simply the amount of calories our body burns other then for digestion and physical activity. Even at a resting state about 60-70% of our necessary daily calorie intake goes toward giving our body the fuel it needs to live. A lot our calories intake goes toward temperature control, whether its trying to cool our body down from external heat or exertion by sweating or by shivering to keep our body warm to counter external cold temperatures.

Either way, calories are simply units of heat that are burned for energy and temperature control (whether for warming or cooling our body), digestion, vital organ activity and fuel to give us the energy we need for daily activities.

When we are constantly in a very temperature controlled environment year round throughout our changing seasons and especially if we're not very active, we will burn fewer calories due to the simple fact that modern air conditioning is taking care of a lot of the workload. So this is one more factor that we can add to the other two that have contributed so much to our obesity epidemic…

1. Diet.

2. Inactivity.

3. Controlled temperatures year round.

(All resulting in far fewer calories burned)!

Our body burns a lot of calories when it goes through the process of expelling extra heat by breaking a sweat, and especially by combating external cold. This gets shifted into high gear when we start shivering to generate heat and you can bet it's burning quite a bit of calories to stimulate either of these actions! Btw even though environmental exposures to heat and cold can stimulate calorie burning and even build our immune systems, when overdone can cause unnecessary stress on and in the body, causing anything from heat stroke to a weakened immune system that makes us more susceptible to the flu etc.

Winter Food Tip: I like to keep some cayenne pepper around to season food, and also some cayenne capsules to take with (at least two) meals a day. I found that it works best when I take the capsules about halfway through my meal. Adding this spiced heat to your diet helps you be a little warmer instead of cold blooded in the winter. This spice can also help you get a sweatier workout when taken 30 min to an hour before the workout. Sweating with a purpose is a great way to help us push out toxins instead of waiting until a fever pushes it out of us, or as we call it breaking a fever.

There are many other benefits of cayenne pepper: research it by doing an Internet search on the following words "Benefits of Cayenne Pepper."

Add this to your daily intake along with beginning and ending the day with some warm/hot water and lemon, and it should add to your body's protective winter arsenal.

HIGH INTENSITY INTERVAL TRAINING (HIIT)

HIIT is simply a way each of us can push ourselves a little harder to build an equal amount of physical strength and cardio conditioning combined with the fat burning effect most of us are after. Most trainers and athletes would look at this as applicable to walking or jogging mixed with intense bouts or sprints that last about 20 seconds. I like to simply apply this as a method of anything you do that is somewhat physical whether work related activity or low intensity exercise combined with anything done at maximum output that revs up your heart rate such as jumping jacks, sprinting etc. and gets your lungs working harder to supply oxygen and nutrients to these working muscles.

This does more then build cardio strength, muscle and endurance, it also excites the system that releases stored energy from inside our fat cells and when we feel this energy hit our system, (we get what many of us know as our 2nd wind) and it does feel good! This usually happens after we have our heart rate revved up for about 20 min and your body recognizes the need for a strong source of energy.

What qualifies as intense movement for one person may not be for another, so you want to go with an amount that is right for you and this is something you want to gradually build up to.

This can even be done with walking.

Try this: after walking for about 3 minutes at a regular pace to warm up, walk really fast for about 1 minute and then slow down for about 30 seconds, then walk really fast for 45 seconds, then 30 seconds slow pace, keep doing drop sets until you get down to a 15 second fast pace for a total of 4 sets. Eventually you will get to where you can do 4 sets of a minute each of fast pace walking. Exercising in this manner has been shown over time to line up proteins in muscle that help deliver fat more efficiently for the mitochondria (energy factory) of our cells to burn as energy.

Whether you choose pushups, jumping jacks or simply grab the side of your desk and do a set of squats, we have many little opportunities to mix in intervals of intense exercise even if it only lasts 30 seconds. This can help us boost our metabolism and give us an edge on meeting our fitness goals!

Even if you're stuck at a desk you can use these same intense exercises to counter the sedentary job, simply by pulling back and doing a full body movement rapidly for a minute. This also pumps more oxygen into your blood helping you to stay alert and energetic instead of sleepy and tired.

Try this: next time you're stuck at your desk, stand up and lean into your desk doing a pushup movement and do this rapidly (for 1 minute), then immediately step back and do some rapid squats (for 1 minute).

We have little snippets of time and opportunities all around us for squeezing in exercise, through our activities of daily living, (ADL's) we just need to do them faster and with greater intensity!

CHRONIC DISEASE IS THE MANIFESTATION OF INFLAMMATION

All major disease has some form of relationship with inflammation, but the two leading causes of death here in the U.S. (Heart Disease and Cancer) are simply inflammation manifested in the form of either of the above and they are projected to be the leading causes of death in developed countries for years to come! Inflammatory reactions are something that comes after a cause and when we have too many of these causes happening to our body over a period of time, these areas it is happening to, will simply build up to a diagnosable state that has a scary name attached to it.

When inflammation gets a name attached to it due to the damage it has done and could continue doing, such as heart disease or cancer, we will have been suffering from it long before the specialist can actually diagnosed what it has or is becoming.

One of the most powerful sources of inflammation is visceral fat. This fat is not the kind that (if kept at reasonable levels) simply gives someone a healthy youthful look and holds reserve energy for low calorie days or periods of starvation, but rather a fat that builds up and surrounds internal organs. It will then release chemicals that produce a slow, smoldering inflammation that in turn gives a fertile environment for incubating a disease. This is not only restricted to ones that are obviously overweight, but it also can also be in a person that appears somewhat thin. The primary difference that I have found with between the two fats subcutaneous fat vs. visceral fat, is that subcutaneous fat causes weight loss frustration visceral fat causes disease. What seems to make a big difference (whatever the size of the person) in the amount of visceral fat a person has, seems to be closely connected with, activity levels, dietary choices and stress levels.

The idea is to avoid the things that actually cause inflammation and to also tip the scale in our favor by doing things that fight inflammation.

There are some things we can do through dour diet to prevent and overcome inflammation.

First the items to really

avoid: sugars, common cooking oils, trans

fats, processed meat, alcohol, refined

grains, artificial food additives. We also should avoid foods that we're sensitive to. These are the foods that cause anything from a fiery reaction to simply making us feel tired, nauseous, headaches and a irritated digestive track.

Foods good for fighting inflammation are: fruits and vegetables, foods rich in omega-3 fatty acids: fish, such as salmon, sardines, tuna and other cold-water fish, nuts, and seeds, especially flax seeds, walnuts, soybeans and olive oil instead of common cooking oils, and anti-inflammatory spices such as: curry powder, cloves and ginger.

An anti-inflammation tool chest: make sure there is adequate fruits, vegetables, healthy fats, oils, herbs, and spices, mixed in your diet and it can really help our body fight it's inflammation battles!

Remember: most teas, onions, garlic, berries, artichokes, and all herbs and spices contain powerful phytonutrients that fight inflammation and protect your body from degenerative diseases. Some of the strongest inflammation fighters in this category are cherries or tart cherry juice, pistachios, and artichokes.

Getting on top of inflammatory issues, and what are causing them, finding the cure, and then incorporating it into our lifestyle for prevention is one of our best means of fighting early death from chronic disease!

Inflammation information exercise: go online and do a search on "Fighting Inflammation."

THE BATTLE OF EXCESS CALORIES

This time of year can be hard to wage a successful war against a build up of excess calories that are either flooding our system or are staring at us everywhere we look! If we would look at food in the same way that we look at fuel for our vehicle, it would make things pretty simple in whether we need fuel or if a refill is not at all necessary. Unlike a vehicle, our fuel tank is expandable and when we overeat, (if we don't burn off these extra calories over the next 3 to 6 hours), our body will simply store this extra fuel inside mini storage cells (fat cells) all over our body, especially if we eat again before this extra is burned off. These extra calories become the energy matter inside our fat cells and this is what causes us to appear overweight.

I have noticed if I eat a lot of heavy food (especially if its toward evening), I can feel adequate fuel in my body up until 2:00 - 4:00

149

pm the next day depending on how much and what type of food it was. A lot of times we mistake hunger for the feeling we get when our body starts getting to the end of a sugar load, this is when you need to wait a little longer and let your body shift its energy source over to burning fat for energy. This is also when you can cash in on the stored calories, but to do so your sugar level has got to drop in your blood.

During the holidays, what I have found that seems to work really well, is creating a calorie deficit (being active and not eating for an extended period) prior to a heavy meal and then doing something to burn off the excess blood sugars about an hour after eating. When I've overdone it one meal, (especially if it was heavy food) I simply skip eating the next meal or go really light, which is exactly what I did the day after Thanksgiving! Part of this is based on my belief that the latest stored energy is the first out over the next 24 hours, and will be readily available if we do not eat anything that is sweet or starchy, this will turn the fat burning process off!

Overeating consecutive heavy meals that are not staggered by light meals that have plenty of fiber is asking for excess weight gain and a colon that has a gradual buildup of old fecal matter.

Getting to know our own body so that we know when it needs food vs. when we need to give it time to clear some food out of our system is important if we want to reduce our weight or keep it in check throughout the holidays!

Sugar locks up the release of energy from fat cells tighter then a lockdown during a prison riot!

A SELF INFLICTED GENOCIDE!

We as a nation have become entirely to comfortable with a reliance on the medical field for our source of health, however when it's not available, it can then be easy to blame it as a source for our un-health, instead of ourselves as victims of our own negligence. I'm sorry if this sounds a little harsh, but once our unhealthy habits as a nation are combined with the coming healthcare bill being implemented, our capability for life extension after years of unhealthy habits will become much harder then it has in the past. A reliance grown on a healthcare system that has been there for every little scratch, bump, lump, bruise, sniffle or nose bleed, I believe will have mass repercussions unless we switch to a personal responsibility mentality for our own health!

The medical field is in place to provide intervention, not prevention, yet we have let our own guard down and have adapted the outlook, of if I get broke I'll get fixed and look to them for vaccinating and medicating strength into our immune system and that of our children through an ever growing list of vaccinations and medications. The medical field and pharmaceutical industry have minted a fortune by a dumbing down of personal responsibility and adding care for people that are relatively healthy and really don't need them and the never ending diagnostic procedures and office visits. Most times, all it would take to get a person's health back on track are the simple basic healthy habits done with consistency. The medical industry is not the master of our health, we are and until we realize that it's a business for them (whether diagnostics, office visits, medications, vaccinations, surgeries, etc.) we will continue risking our health while in the pursuit of it!

  This is an example of just one of the things that could happen and is a part of what I believe is the coming tsunami: we have a growing epidemic of diabetes on the horizon, which can lead to many more of us needing dialysis due to kidney failures caused by diabetes. If we need 3 treatments a week (to filter the toxins out of our blood), but because of the provider getting more business then they can keep up with, (we are instead scheduled for only 2 weekly treatments), we will have more toxins left in our body for longer and the toxins will be doing what they do best, generating chronic and infectious disease.

I was watching the documentary on CNBC, "Fat and Fatter; Inside the Obesity Epidemic" and it really struck me when the lady (that weighed 500 pounds was getting one of her 3 times a week dialysis treatments), told the overweight young girl interviewing her that she would die within a week if she missed her dialysis treatments. Her advice was simple, you need to take responsibility because you may not have access to the same care I do. Though people abuse usage of the healthcare system, when we need it and we cannot access it, we can die rapidly without these life-extending procedures the medical profession provides!

We add to this by our inactive, high stress lives, and eating processed food and drink that are loaded with sugar, sodium, starches, preservatives, and chemical taste enhancers!

The average American eats 29 pounds of French fries, 23 pounds of pizza, 24 pounds of ice cream and consumes 53 gallons of soda, 150 pounds of refined sugars, 24 pounds of artificial sweeteners, 2.736 pounds of processed salt and 90,700 mg of caffeine per year.

If we could only have the one car we own now for the rest of our life, would we take care of it any differently then we do now?

CAFFEINE AND SUGAR, A POISONOUS COCKTAIL!

Americans eat 150 pounds of refined sugars, 24 pounds of artificial sweeteners, and 90,700 mg of caffeine per year.

I will say it makes me a little uncomfortable talking about this, especially when its about someone's morning-hug-in-a-mug, but its a combination I feel is important to address due to the poisonous physiological effect it has in our body when consumed together.

We have been consuming loads of starchy, sugary caffeinated products combined with a huge decrease in activity and the devastating combinational effect is very obvious (in the distorted shapes and massive onslaught of diabetes)! If we believe in cause and effect and simply trace lines backwards from the effects we can pretty easily find the culprit(s).

Example: high sugar, high fat, caffeinated diets combined with low levels of activity = obesity & chronic disease.

Synergy, (the amplified effect) between products such as supplements, medications, chemicals and foods whether good or bad is something that really interests me. Some products when used together have a stronger effect then they do by themselves and this can be good, but when products are combined that do not go well together, it can have a bad effect on a person or the environment.

Example: If you mix certain household chemicals together, the synergy can range from putting off a toxic gas to exploding!

However in the case of combining caffeine and sugar its much more subtle, and may take a little while before the damages really start surfacing. We already have one strike against it due to the fact that most of these caffeinated sugar drinks and desserts do not have soluble fiber in them to slow the sugar absorption down (such as in a fruit) so besides dumping sugar almost directly into our blood, we also escalate the whole process by adding caffeine! Our body recognizes an elevation of blood sugar and will then produce insulin to carry this sugar (energy) to our cells; however, caffeine causes temporary insulin insensitivity thus blocking this energy uptake.

The best I can figure out on this is that if the reaction of caffeine is to cause insulin insensitivity, it would mean one thing to me; caffeine has a purpose of releasing energy, not its uptake, causing us to potentially have released energy from our fat cells entering our system. This combination plus the extra sugar load from the caffeinated drink can be really bad if we're not doing something during this time to burn off the extra blood sugars.

Insulin tries to push sugar into our cells (this gives us a thing we know as a sugar rush) but when the caffeine has pounced on our cell receptors it will cause them to block the insulin from bringing in the sugar. This causes the pancreas to crank out even more insulin, to try to force the uptake despite the caffeine, and this can then potentially cause insulin resistance which helps wear out our pancreas leading to a dependence on added insulin to combat diabetes.

 I believe however that an exception can be made,

when caffeine and sugar are combined prior to a time period that we are going to be very physically active. The devastating effects most likely are when combined with inactivity or a sedentary lifestyle.

 Take away: Sugar and caffeine should not be mixed, especially before periods of inactivity or low levels of activity!

Artificial sweeteners (such as Sweet n Low, Equal and Splenda) are bad on your thyroid (the organ that regulates our metabolism). They are also neurotoxic causing an inflammatory response from our body, leading to a release of cortisol, which in turn will signal our body to retain belly fat.

Coffee and Tea have many heath benefits by themselves. Opt for extra cream and a little stevia.

Lets make this easier to do by asking ourselves, does this sweet poison taste as good to my body as it did to my mouth?

IS IT GUNS OR THE BRAIN THAT DICTATES THE OUTCOME?

 The tasks computers carry out are largely dependent on how their software is programmed. Without the software programming that the programmer coded into the software the computer would simply be a bunch of hardware that can do absolutely nothing. However, sometimes we allow viruses to slip in that are not good for the brain of our computer(s) and it will corrupt the original programming.

 I was not planning to write about this, but it's absolutely hard for me to think beyond the subject of mental health after what happened Friday in Connecticut. This was the most heinous act that I have seen or heard of since the slaughter of the Amish school children in Lancaster County, PA in 2006 ages 6-13.

Being in the field of fitness and nutrition I am a strong believer in looking not so much at the problem itself, then in trying to figure out where the root system of the problem is getting fed. If you starve off this supply line to the problem, it has no choice but to die. Unfortunately we have gotten to where we like to medicate and suppress the symptoms allowing many in the medical profession to keep the problem alive thus creating massive sustainable windfall profits for the pharmaceutical industry through their SSRI prescribed brain drugs!

Wall Street Journal 9/21/2012: There are enough people killed each week by medical error to fill 4 jumbo jets. Do we really want to use these drugs just because the medical field is saying this is what we need? Lets do our own research before subjecting our brain or that of our children to chemical control.

I would love to see the medical prescription history of these people and here's the reason; when we grow a person's brain dependency on behavioral medicine while they are a child, we are as a person, family or society then subjected to this child when he or she becomes an adult, to acknowledge themselves as a mentally imbalanced person without drugs, (I'm sure this doesn't feel good to accept as a young adult). So how many of these children will potentially grow up and decide to suddenly no longer take the medicine(s) that treats their neurological disorders?

We live in a society that has purposely been trying to extract reference to God out, along with smirking in the face of Christian morals and in turn has been feeding brains with control drugs, programming them with violent video games and movies and when this is combined with known neurotoxins (brain/nerve poisons) in our vaccinations, medications and diet, and to not look at these as a potential feed for the root system of what happens in brain development and to think that we can just throw brain control drugs at all our children's behavioral issues without the potential of effecting brain development is just plain stupid.

Politically people are jumping on gun control issues whether in opposition or in defense of current gun laws, and probably many of those in opposition would at the same time take a valiant stand in defense of their alcohol the drug that has probably destroyed more people's lives, health, marriages, families, and businesses then illegal drugs and guns combined. So my question is this, are we as a country going to be able to figure out if the vehicles, guns, knives, hammers and box cutters cause intentional death or is it the body that houses a brain that has become void of good? This is not a case of which come first, the chicken or the egg. Its simple, a normal functioning body will do the directives of the brain whether good or bad and when the software of our brain gets warped anything from our health to physical actions inflicted to ourselves or the ones around us will suffer. Matter of fact, when the brain gets turned off the rest of us will start shutting down almost like the Energizer Bunny without its battery.

We probably all have a little bit of crazy, a little bit of bad and a little bit of potential psychosis (or loss of contact with reality) in us, but our means of suppression of this side of us and a further development of our good and moral side that is instilled in each of us like a compass and is key to the bad side not taking control of our lives and thus our actions.

HEALTH TIPS: A YEAR IN REVIEW

 I thought it might be of benefit to highlight some of the main things these articles in this volume have covered...

1. Aging = Oxidation & Oxidation = Aging! Our body works like an energy factory and if we don't help it to release its smoke, the toxins will build up and cause problems. Water, sweat, antioxidants from fruits and vegetables, and our waste elimination system are like our smoke stack that helps us release and cleanse out these toxins that cause aging and disease.

 2. Slowing metabolism, muscle, skeletal and cardiovascular weaknesses, often has more to do with muscle loss (atrophy) then with aging. The main cause of this is inactivity. Our body builds what we tell it to, but also shrinks what we tell it to, by either activity or inactivity and a dietary intake that is either made up of foods that build our body and health or one that makes it unhealthy and out of shape. Our dietary intake and activity largely dictates the outcome, whether our health or shape!

3. Intermittent Fasting (IF) skipping food for 18-24 hours will trick the body into switching over to burning fat as an energy source. Going longer then this can make our body think it's starving, it will then start burning muscle for fuel to slow our metabolism down.

4. Health & Fitness Goals are about 75% dependent on what we eat and drink!

The foods we surround ourselves with are what we will start to look and feel like!

5. Eat local grown fruits & vegetables whenever you can these are the best sources of multi-vitamins and minerals! Limit food and drink that have multiple ingredients in them. Eat many different foods for a variety of nutrients, fats, proteins, carbohydrates, vitamins and minerals, our body will pick and pull what it needs.

6. We are Never too Old for Exercise & Fitness: when we strengthen muscles, tendons, ligaments and bones, we increase capability for easy movement and mobility thus increasing the economy of movement as we get older which in turn increases quality of life.

7. The Doctor is not a source for health and prevention: they know very little about this~ the medical field is a field that specializes in intervention, not prevention!

8. We die the fastest without oxygen (within minutes), so why breathe filthy oxygen (such as cigarette smoke) into our lungs, lining them with soot? Water is 2nd in line, (we'll die in 3 days without it). We need water to flush toxic waste out of our cells and bodies, so drink plenty and drink it pure without sugars, carbonation, and chemicals! Food is 3rd on the list, we are what we eat so lets make so that our body has good building material to work with!

9. Obesity is the one thing most all-chronic diseases have in common.

10. The food cocaine's of the American diet (salt and sugar) have distorted the shape and health of America. Preparing our own food puts us back in control of this!

11. Keeping Our Body More Alkaline and Less Acidic will make our body less friendly to disease!

12. A Healthy Immune System is Your Vaccination against dependence on the Healthcare System.

13. Chronic Disease is simply the Manifestation of Inflammation. Making sure there are adequate fruits, vegetables, healthy fats, oils, herbs, and spices, mixed in our diet can really help our body fight its inflammation battles!

14. Follow a heavy meal (high calories) with one or two light calorie meals. It will help lower the calories in our body so that we won't store them in our fat cells. The energy matter inside our cells is what makes us appear fat not the cell itself.

15. You do not have to have a gym or gym equipment to exercise; rapid bodyweight movement increases resistance thus building your muscle, strength and metabolism.

16. Caffeine and sugar are a really bad combination when consumed at the same time. The caffeine attaches to our cells receptors temporarily blocking sugar from entering the cells, thus blocking it in the blood causing blood sugar problems.

17. Eat foods rich in soluble fiber to lower cholesterol and to slow sugar absorption from digesting food into your bloodstream. Eating foods rich in insoluble fiber help us recognize when we have consumed enough food.

18. Look up health, fitness, and nutritional questions by simply typing in any question you have on the Internet behind your question. Any of the above list that you want to expand upon, simply phrase a question about it and you can research it as far as you want to go with it. This is my way of teaching people how to fish.

19. The brain is the control center of the body, when this is no longer healthy or stops working, we start shutting down, so lets learn what we can to keep it healthy, active and keep bad stuff from getting into our brain and controlling our voluntary and involuntary actions.

20. In 90-120 days our blood supply is replaced by a new blood supply - in approximately 6 months our soft tissue is replaced by new tissue - and in approximately a 12-month period everything all the way down to our bone and tooth enamel is replaced by a new cell generation. Though its a mutation from the prior generation of cells, we have the opportunity to make the next year's generation of cells healthier simply by sticking to the few basic healthy habits and by doing them with consistency,

1. Clean Air

2. Plenty Water

3. Balanced Diet.

4. Deep Rest.

5. Stay Active.

6. Sunshine.

7. Get rid of your stress daily.

Your body is designed to be a survival machine with an Internal Doctor that works 24-7-365 so whatever our starting point is, lets give it the tools it needs to do its job!!!

I wish you all the best in health & Fitness~ Wade Yoder

About the author

Wade Yoder has been in the health and fitness club business since 1991 and is a weekly health and fitness columnist for 5 Middle, Georgia newspapers with over 160 published articles since 2012.
He owns and operates Valley Athletic Club in Fort Valley, Georgia

Master Trainer certifications:

Fitness Trainer - Fitness Nutrition

Fitness Therapy - Strength and Conditioning

Senior Fitness & Youth Fitness

www.ingramcontent.com/pod-product-compliance
Lightning Source LLC
Chambersburg PA
CBHW072011290526

45787CB00013B/318